Endorsements for *A Stra[ing Understanding] of Mental Health Problems*

What people said about the first edition:

'An accessible look at complex issues that empowers the reader to start thinking for themselves. A refreshing antidote to the simplistic and pessimistic biomedical model.'
Jacqui Dillon, activist, writer, speaker and former Chair, Hearing Voices Network

'Brilliantly engaging, understandable and thoughtful… will equip service users, carers and professionals alike with empowering knowledge.'
Tony Morrison, Professor of Clinical Psychology, University of Manchester

'Perfect for the non-professional. Bought this book while studying level 2 counselling. It's well written and easy to understand, without all the technical jargon.'
Online reviewer

'What causes mental health problems? Lots of things combining together. This book describes them, clearly and systematically, and how they interact.'
David Kingdon, Emeritus Professor of Mental Health Care Delivery, University of Southampton

A STRAIGHT TALKING INTRODUCTION TO THE CAUSES OF MENTAL HEALTH PROBLEMS

JOHN READ & PETE SANDERS

REVISED SECOND EDITION

PCCS BOOKS

First edition published 2010
This edition published 2022

PCCS Books Ltd
Wyastone Business Park
Wyastone Leys
Monmouth
NP25 3SR
UK

Tel +44 (0)1600 891509
contact@pccs-books.co.uk
www.pccs-books.co.uk

© John Read and Pete Sanders

All rights reserved. No part of this publication may be reproduced, stored in a retrieval system, transmitted or utilised in any form by any means, electronic, mechanical, photocopying or recording or otherwise without permission in writing from the publishers.

No responsibility for loss caused to any individual or organisation acting on or refraining from action as a result of the material in the publication can be accepted by PCCS Books or the authors.

The authors have asserted their right to be identified as the authors of this work in accordance with the Copyright, Designs and Patents Act 1988.

A Straight Talking Introduction to the Causes of Mental Health Problems
(second edition)

British Library Cataloguing in Publication Data.
A catalogue record for this book is available from the British Library

ISBNs
paperback – 978 1 915220 19 6
epub – 978 1 915220 20 2

Cover design by Jason Anscomb
Printed in the UK by Severn, Gloucester

A Straight Talking Introduction to the Causes of Mental Health Problems (second edition)

Contents

	Introducing the *Straight Talking Introductions* series *Richard Bentall and Pete Sanders*	*vii*
1	Our beliefs and values	*1*
2	A brief history of beliefs about the causes of human distress	*15*
3	The 20th century and beyond: the illness model	*27*
4	Do diagnoses help us understand causes?	*49*
5	Public opinion: depression is caused by depressing things happening	*59*
6	Is the public right? What does the research say about the causes of mental health problems?	*69*
7	Psychological theories: how events operate on us to create problems	*88*
8	Putting things together: formulating depression	*113*
9	2010–2022 and looking to the future: a call for action	*126*
	References	*141*
	Further reading and resources	*156*
	Name index	*165*
	Subject index	*169*

Pete © John Read

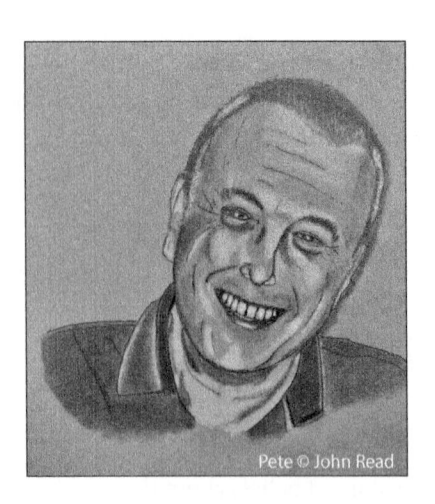

Dedication

Pete died in February this year. Even though we all knew he was living on borrowed time because of his precarious heart condition, his disappearance from our world was still a shock and has left a gaping hole. Thank you, Maggie, for gathering us, friends and family, together in Hereford to share stories of this lovely, inspiring, warm, strong-willed man.

Pete will live on in our hearts and memories, and, of course, in all the wonderful books he has nurtured into life, including his own. I am happy to have my name on one of them.

Goodbye Pete. Thanks for showing us what a life well lived looks like. We love you.

John Read
September 2022

About the authors

Dr John Read has worked in the UK, USA and New Zealand for 20 years as a clinical psychologist. He is currently Professor of Clinical Psychology at the University of East London. He has edited several books, including *Models of Madness* (2013). He has been editor of the research journal *Psychosis: Psychological, social and integrative approaches* since 2009. John is Chair of the International Institute for Psychiatric Drug Withdrawal (www.iipdw.org).

Pete Sanders worked as a volunteer at 'Off The Record', Newcastle-upon Tyne, in 1972 before completing a degree in psychology at the university there, and then the Postgraduate Diploma in Counselling at Aston University. He practised as a counsellor, educator and clinical supervisor for more than 30 years. He wrote, co-wrote and edited numerous books, chapters and papers on many aspects of counselling, psychotherapy and mental health, and in particular developing person-centred theory, the politics of counselling and psychotherapy, and the demedicalisation of distress. He was a pre-therapy contact work trainer, trustee of Open Door Counselling Birmingham and patron of the Soteria Network UK. Pete died in February 2022, before this book was updated in this second edition.

....

Co-editor with Pete Sanders of this series, Richard Bentall is Professor of Clinical Psychology at the University of Sheffield and has previously held chairs at Liverpool, Manchester, and Bangor universities. He is a Fellow of the British Psychological Society and of the British Academy. His research has focused on the cognitive and emotional mechanisms involved in psychotic symptoms such as hallucinations and delusions, and also examined why social risk factors (for example childhood adversities) provoke the cognitive and emotional changes that lead to these symptoms. He has also conducted clinical trials of novel psychological treatments for psychosis.

Acknowledgements

John Read would like to acknowledge the many users of mental health services who have trusted him enough to share their understandings of the causes of their difficulties.

In his acknowledgements in the first edition, Pete Sanders wrote:
Pete Sanders owes a great debt to all of the patients and some of the staff he met in institutions in the late 1960s and early 1970s. Their struggles to maintain and, where possible, celebrate human dignity in a plainly crazy system continue to help him make choices in life.

Introducing the *Straight Talking Introductions* series

What are mental health problems?

Much of what is written and spoken about emotional distress or mental health problems implies that they are illnesses. This can lead us all too easily to believe that we no longer have to think about mental health problems, because illness is best left to doctors. They are the illness experts, and psychiatrists are the doctors who specialise in mental illness. This series of books is different because we don't think that all mental health problems should automatically be regarded as illnesses.

If mental health problems aren't necessarily illnesses, it means that the burden of responsibility for distress in our lives should not be shouldered entirely by doctors and psychiatrists. All citizens have a responsibility, however small, in creating a world where everyone has a decent opportunity to live a fulfilling life. This is a contentious idea, but one that we want to advance, alongside the dominant medical view.

Rather than accept that the ways of understanding and solutions to mental health problems are 'owned' by the medical profession, we will take a good look at alternatives that involve the users of psychiatric services, their carers, families, friends and other 'ordinary people' taking control of their own lives, and that means all of us. One of the tools required in order to become active in mental health issues, whether your own or other people's, is knowledge. This series of books is a starting point for anyone who wants to know more about mental health.

How these books are written

Information

We want these books to be understandable, so we use everyday language wherever possible. The books could have been almost completely jargon-free, but we thought that including some technical and medical terms would be helpful. Most doctors, psychiatrists and psychologists use the medical model of mental illness and manuals to help them diagnose mental health problems. The medical model and the diagnostic manuals use a particular set of terms to describe what doctors think of as 'conditions'. Although these words aren't very good at describing individual people's experiences, they are used a lot in psychiatric and psychological services, so we thought it would be helpful to define these terms as we went along and use them in a way that might help readers understand what the professionals mean. We don't expect that psychiatrists and psychologists and others working in mental health services will stop using medical terminology (although we think it would be respectful for them to drop it when talking to their patients and their families), so these books should help you get used to and learn *their* language.

The books also contain resources for further learning. As well as lists of books, websites and organisations at the end of the book, there are references. These will not be important to everyone, but they do tell the reader where information – a claim about effectiveness, an argument for or against, or a quotation – has come from, so you can follow it up if you wish.

Being realistic and reassuring

Our aim is to be realistic – neither overly optimistic nor pessimistic. Things are nearly always more complicated than we would like them to be. Honest evaluations of mental health problems, of what might cause them, of what can help and of what the likely outcome might be, are, like so much in life, somewhere in between. For the vast majority of people, it would be wrong to say that they have an illness from which they will never recover. But it would be equally wrong to say that they will be completely unchanged by the distressing thoughts and feelings they are having. Life is an accumulation of experiences. There is almost certainly no pill, or any other treatment for that matter, that will take us back to 'how we were before'. There are many things we can do (and we look at lots of them in this series), in collaboration with doctors, psychiatrists, psychologists and counsellors, and, indeed, everyone working in mental health services, with the help of our friends and family, or on our own, that stand a good chance of helping us feel better and build a constructive life, with hope for the future.

Of course, we understand that the experiences dealt with in these books can sometimes be so overwhelming, confusing and terrifying that people will try to escape from them by withdrawing, going mad or even trying to kill themselves. This happens when our usual coping strategies fail us. We accept that killing oneself is, in some circumstances, a rational act – that, for the person in question, it can make a lot of sense. Nonetheless, we believe that much of the distress that underpins such an extreme course of action, from which there can be no turning back, is avoidable. For this reason, all of the books in this series point towards realistic hope and recovery.

Debates

There is no single convenient answer to many of the most important questions explored in these books. No matter how badly we might wish for a simple answer, what we have is a series of debates, or arguments, more like, between stakeholders, and there are many stakeholders whose voices demand space in these books. We use the word 'stakeholders' here because service users, carers, friends, family, doctors, psychologists, psychiatrists, nurses and other healthcare workers, scientists in drug companies, therapists and, indeed, all citizens, have a stake in how our society understands and deals with problems of mental health. It is simultaneously big business and intimately personal, and many things in between. As we go along, we try to explain how someone's stake in distress (including our own, where we can see it), whether professional or personal, can influence their experience and judgement.

While we want to present competing (sometimes opposing) viewpoints, we don't want to leave the reader high and dry to evaluate complicated debates on their own. We will try to present reasonable conclusions that might point in certain directions for personal action. Above all, though, we believe that knowledge is power and that the better informed you are, even though the information might be conflicting, the more able you will be to make sound decisions.

It's also useful to be reminded that the professionals involved in helping distressed people are themselves caught in the same flow of conflicting information. It is their *job*, however, to interpret it in our service, so that the best solutions are available to as many people as possible. You may have noticed that the word 'best' brings with it certain challenges, not least defining what we mean when we use this term. Perhaps 'the best' means the most effective? However, even using words like 'effective' doesn't completely clear up the puzzle. An effective treatment for an employer could be the one that returns a member of staff to work quickly; for a parent, it could be one that makes their child feel happier and calmer. For the government or the NHS, or someone running a private healthcare business, 'effective' might mean 'cost-effective'. This brings us to evidence.

Evidence

Throughout these books there will be material that we will present as 'evidence'. This is one of the most contentious terms to be found in this series. One person's evidence is another person's fanciful mythology and yet another person's oppressive propaganda. Nevertheless, the term crops up increasingly in everyday settings, most relevantly when we hear of 'evidence-based practice'. The idea behind this term is that the treatments psychologists and psychiatrists offer should be those that 'work'. Crudely put, there should be some evidence that, say, talking about problems or taking a prescribed drug actually helps people feel better. We encounter a real problem, however, when trying to evaluate this evidence, as the books in this series will demonstrate. We will try not to discount any 'evidence' out of hand, but we will critically evaluate it, and we will do this with a bias towards scientific evaluation.

The types of evidence that will be covered in these books, along with their positive and negative points, include the following.

Research methods, numbers and statistics

On the one hand, the logic of most research is simple, but on the other hand, the way things have to be arranged to avoid bias in the results can lead to a perplexing system of measurements. Even the experts lose the sense of it, sometimes. We'll try to explain the logic of studies, but almost certainly leave out the details. You can look these up yourself if you wish.

The books in this series look at research into a wide range of issues relating to mental health problems, including the experience of distress, what is known about the causes of problems, and their prevention and treatment. Different research methods are appropriate for each of these areas, so we will be looking at different types of research as we go along. We say this now because many readers may be most familiar with studies into the *effective treatments* of distress, and we want to emphasise that there are many other credible and valid sources of essential information about distress that are sometimes overlooked.

You may have come across the idea that some research methods are 'better' than others – that they constitute a 'gold standard'. In the case of research into the effectiveness of different treatments, the gold standard is usually considered to be randomised controlled trials (RCTs). In simple terms, RCTs are complex (and often very expensive) experiments in which a group of individuals who all suffer from the same problem are allocated randomly to a treatment (such as a drug or a form of talking therapy) or a 'control' treatment (at its simplest, no treatment at all, or a dummy pill or 'placebo') to test if the treatment works. We are not necessarily convinced that RCTs always *are* the best way of proving the effectiveness of different treatments, but they are, currently, the method given most credence by the bodies that control funding and what it is spent on, such as (in England) the National Institute for Health and Care Excellence (NICE) – so we need to understand them.

Before it is accepted by academics and clinicians, research must be written up and published in a journal that asks independent people to read it, to make sure that it is *bona fide* and that no glaring mistakes have been made. In recent years, a number of high-profile academics and scientific commentators have drawn attention to possible problems with this system of quality control. This series of books is not the place to deal with these arguments, but where they impinge on the evidence in a particular area, we will make sure it is highlighted.

Personal experience

Personal experience is an important source of evidence, to the extent that, nowadays, people who have suffered debilitating psychiatric distress are sometimes called 'experts by experience'. Personal stories provide an essential counterbalance to the impersonal numbers and statistics often found in research projects such as RCTs. While not everyone is average, by definition most people are. Balancing the average results obtained from RCTs with some personal stories helps complete the picture and is now widely accepted, to the extent that it has given birth to the new field of 'survivor research'.

Understanding contexts

Widening our view to include people's families and lives and the cultural, economic, social and political settings in which we live completes the picture. Mental health problems are connected to the conditions in which we all live, just as much as they are connected to our biology. From the start, we want readers to know that, if there is one message or model that these books are trying to get across, it is that problems in mental health are more often than not the result of complex events in the environments in which we live and our reactions to them. These reactions can also be influenced by our biology and the way we have learned to think and feel. Hopefully, these books will help disentangle the puzzle of distress and provide positive suggestions and hope for us all, whether we work in the system, currently have mental health problems ourselves or are caring for or friends with someone who has.

We hope that readers of these books will feel empowered by what they learn and thereby feel more able to get the best out of mental health services. It would be wonderful if our efforts, directly or indirectly, influence the development of services that effectively address the emotional, social and practical needs of people with mental health problems.

Richard Bentall
Pete Sanders
2021

Chapter 1
Our beliefs and values

Our thinking about the causes of mental health problems is, like our ideas about anything, shaped primarily by our life experiences. Although everything that follows in this book is supported by research findings (some of which we will describe, as examples), different authors with different lives and different beliefs and motives could produce a very different book.

For example, John always starts his first lecture to a new student intake with a short personal history to show where his beliefs – or, as some would say, 'biases' – come from. This is his attempt to demonstrate that, despite all the research studies we will be covering later, everyone's beliefs about what causes human distress, madness and so on are really still just beliefs. And those beliefs come largely from our life experiences, from the beliefs of other people whom we trust and respect, and various other 'subjective' rather than 'objective' sources. Our backgrounds go some way to explain our beliefs about the causes of mental health problems.

John writes:

Looking back, I now realise that one of the reasons I went into mental health work was that it was reassuring to know there were people more screwed up than me. At the time, however, I simply thought I wanted to help people. I guess I also preferred the helper role to the helpee role.

Perhaps because I was part-way bonkers myself or could at least understand why one might want to kill oneself, I seemed to be quite good at connecting to people in extreme states of distress, despair and confusion. I was more fascinated than scared (but sometimes only just) when people heard voices I couldn't hear or had weird beliefs about people being out to get them. I was sufficiently paranoid myself in those years that, when the psychiatrist in the New York hospital where I was working as a nursing aide complimented me on my ability to build relationships with even the most 'psychotic' people, and asked me how I did it, I was so convinced that he was making fun of me that I slithered away to cry in the staff room. A kind nurse used her own considerable skills to convince me I had been wrong and that she too thought I was pretty good at the job.

Anyway, here are just three of the stories about how I came to believe that 'bad things happening' is usually sufficient explanation for 'mental health problems' and why asking the person concerned what they think is going on can be better than thinking you've explained something by throwing a diagnostic label, or a biological theory, at it.

He had been on the ward for three days without opening his eyes. No mean feat. The doctors had been trying to figure this out, but 'eye-closed behaviour' just wasn't anywhere to be found in the diagnostic manual. One night, about 2 a.m., I asked him, more from boredom than clinical judgement, why he kept his eyes shut. He immediately opened them, put his face uncomfortably close to mine, and said, 'It's about fucking time one of you idiots asked me that!' He then explained to me that he had been put in the hospital, against his will, to get 'insight' and that's what he had been doing!

Just before my very first chance to help run the weekly group therapy session, an older woman approached me to explain that she wouldn't be talking in the group because she thought that whatever she had said in the past in the group had always been turned into a 'symptom' and used against her. She explained that she didn't want me to be offended by her silence. (I think she could see I was nervous.) After the group, I retreated to the staff team where the patients' performance in the group was evaluated.

There, the woman's not speaking was interpreted by the rest of the team as a sure sign of her paranoia.

I was 'specialing' a teenage girl. This meant being locked in with her in the 'quiet room' (the noisiest place on the ward) to make sure she didn't try, again, to kill herself by smashing her head into the wall. She hadn't spoken for weeks. A 'catatonic schizophrenic'. Having had no training, I tried: 'It's okay if you don't want to talk, but if you do that's okay too.' She didn't. She said nothing for the whole two hours. The next day we were locked in again. This time she started to speak but stopped after just one word: 'My …' The next day she said 'father'.

Okay, I thought, I can do this – one word a day. The next day, however, she reverted to silence for the two hours. The next day she said 'me'. Now we had 'My father… me.' The missing word, I learned later from a family meeting, was 'raped'.

It all seemed rather simple to me. The people in the hospital had had bad, sometimes horrific, experiences and were reacting to them in perfectly understandable ways. But they were only understandable if you knew what had happened.

And they will only tell you what has happened if you are genuinely interested and show that you will listen. If, on the other hand, you start from the premise that they have some terrible illness or are irreversibly mad and that what they say is just a symptom of that illness, disorder or madness, then you can't easily establish the relationship necessary to be told what has happened. This becomes a self-fulfilling prophecy. Without knowing what has gone on in a person's life, and how they have made sense of it for themselves, some people's ways of coping with it all can indeed look a bit strange – even totally crazy.

The diagnoses that the psychiatrists and psychologists spent so much time deciding on, and the theories about genetics and brain dysfunction that always seemed to accompany them, never made much sense to me. They always, right from the start in that first job in New York, seemed to create the illusion of an explanation while explaining nothing at all. I remember asking a psychiatrist how he knew that a woman we were discussing had 'schizophrenia'. 'Because she has the symptoms of schizophrenia,' he replied. 'How do you know they are the symptoms of schizophrenia?' I persisted. The psychiatrist answered, 'Because they are the things that schizophrenics do.' The explanation was accompanied by such an air of certainty that there seemed no point continuing the conversation. I liked this particular psychiatrist very much. He was caring and intelligent, and very supportive of this naïve 22-year-old, despite all my silly questions. But there seemed, to me, to be a major flaw in his circular thinking.

As I progressed through my training as a clinical psychologist and numerous jobs as a psychologist and manager of mental health services, my beliefs about the causes of human distress have been repeatedly reinforced. They have been further reinforced by my studies and my own research since I re-entered academia in 1994.

Of course, it is quite possible that I am guilty of precisely what I often accuse overly biological psychiatrists of doing. Perhaps, like Simon and Garfunkel, I just 'see what I want to see and disregard the rest'. Certainly for years I was vehemently 'opposed' to any theories about brains and genes – having seen the damage done to people's lives by these theories minimising, or ignoring altogether, the social causes of distress and despair. So I try to be honest about my biases. I think this is better than pretending that, in the difficult task of answering the question 'What causes mental health problems?', it is possible to be completely scientific and 'objective'.

Pete writes:

In my mid-to-late teens I got successive holiday jobs in both a local psychiatric hospital and (as it was known then) a 'hospital for the mentally subnormal'. As a 17-year-old from a family with no real exposure to mental health problems, my first day was like a descent into hell. I was overwhelmed by the sights, sounds and smells of the place. I had no way of understanding any of it – it was profoundly disturbing. Nevertheless, I knuckled down and got on with the job, which was to be a 'nursing assistant'. I did everything from helping patients with everyday care such as feeding, shaving, washing and going to the toilet through to sitting on someone while they were injected with paraldehyde. I am still haunted by the smell.

When I was 18, my father died suddenly of a heart attack, three weeks before my A-level exams. He was just 48 years old. I was a pretty happy-go-lucky lad until this happened – it was my first experience of real loss in my life. The family (my 14-year-old brother, my Mom and me) were close, and my Dad had always been a very 'hands-on' father.

Shocking and completely unexpected, Dad's death completely knocked the stuffing out of me. I really didn't know how to carry on, and our wider family (uncles, aunts, grandmothers and so on) were also profoundly affected because Dad was the youngest of five. On the day of the funeral, just after the service at the crematorium, my uncle took me to one side and told me that I was the man of the family now. He told me that, in order to make my Dad proud, I must look after my Mom and brother, pass my A-levels and go to university. It seemed quite reasonable at the time. I reckoned I was doing quite well really.

My dad died a minute or two after midnight. At the hospital, Mom and I were ushered into a waiting room and shortly a pleasant nurse came in and said, 'I'm sorry, we've lost him, Mrs Sanders', while she quickly pressed a tablet into my hand (I was sobbing by then) and said, 'This will help.' It was Librium (chlordiazepoxide, a benzodiazepine tranquilliser).

From then on, I was on autopilot, chemically insulated from grief, and did exactly what my uncle said I must. I still can't remember the next three weeks, or the exams, or the rest of the summer, and it wasn't till I got to university to study psychology and sought some solace in drugs that I hit the ground hard. I later realised that I had suffered a psychotic episode. The GP at the university health centre was an incredibly kind man who clearly thought he had a talent for psychiatry, and I later learned he was renowned for not referring people to specialist services if he thought he didn't really have to. In my case, this was a godsend. He listened to me ramble (sometimes very late into the night) and prescribed some antipsychotic meds, but stopped them pretty soon when he thought I was doing okay. He helped me manage my own experiences (sometimes not too well, and sometimes I needed help), and it was his encouragement to take control of my life that restored me to a reasonable balance. Some people might think that he was the father to me that I was missing so much. Who knows? In my ramblings with him, I began to put some pieces together about my buried experiences of grief and loss, but it took time – most of the rest of my time as an undergraduate.

As I wrestled with terrible anxiety and very frightening strange thoughts, I remembered my time as a nursing assistant and realised that another GP might have had me committed to a mental hospital. I believed I had had a very lucky escape. All of this made me an avid consumer of literature on psychology and psychiatry. And, as I learned more in the early 1970s, I went to antipsychiatry meetings and decided that I wanted to help other people in the way the university health centre doctor had helped me. I thought, based on my own experience, that people should be helped to self-manage and understand their experiences, not have them chemically suppressed. It might take time, but, with luck and kindness, it leads to a lasting healing.

So, one of your tasks, as a reader of this book, is to remember that your authors come to the issues with a set of clearly formed opinions. We suspect, however, that you do too. The difference is that you are open-minded enough to be reading the book, in hope of some new ideas, rather than writing it in hope of sharing ideas that have been held by the authors for decades.

Regardless of what you may want to believe about the relative importance of personal histories and scientific evidence, the research literature about the causes of mental health problems is a bit like the Bible, in two ways. First, most of it is disputed – whatever it says – mostly because science progresses by trying to prove hypotheses wrong and the ensuing debate is expected to take us closer to the truth. This makes life very interesting if you are a scientist, but it's not so good if you or someone close to you is suffering mental distress and you want answers you can trust – answers that will last and will not be superseded next year by new evidence; in short, answers that will help.

Second, the range of evidence is so broad and diverse, and in places downright contradictory, that you can almost always find stuff to support your own beliefs. We think that mental health researchers who believe they are immune to this sort of bias – i.e. who believe that they are purely objective scientists – are kidding themselves. Naturally, if you have suffered distress or have cared for a friend or relative who has suffered, these experiences will shape your beliefs. And, just as surely, those of us whose job involves caring for people who are suffering distress will have both personal and professional beliefs (we like to call them 'theories').

If we look back at our lives, we can develop all sorts of theories about what caused us to be the way we were as children, teenagers and adults. This is especially so if we have suffered any kind of hardship, bullying, emotional, physical and/or sexual abuse or other trauma. We guess every one of you reading this book could come up with a list of childhood, teenage and adult events, good and bad, that you think had an effect on the sort of person you were then and are today. All these experiences will contribute to your understanding of distress, madness, mental illness, or whatever term you use to describe it, and will even determine those terms.

Ways of thinking about causes

This book is about possible causes of what are often called 'mental illnesses'. This sentence takes us straight away to an important issue. Our thinking about people's different mental experiences as 'illnesses' is only one of many possible ways of understanding what might be happening. Yet it is a way that has become so natural to many of us that we think it is a fact about the world. We are inviting the readers of this book to try to step back from these assumptions about what is true and take a new look. Why? In the first place, human experiences are extremely variable and complex. This points to the causes being equally complex, however comforting and convenient it would be if they were simpler. Starting out thinking that different experiences are symptoms of illnesses will artificially narrow our search. We would tend to simply find what we are looking for, rather than what might actually be there.

Second, we have to accept that our understanding of just about everything in the world, however expert we are in a subject, is an unfinished work in progress. Current explanations of mental experiences are the best guesses we have at the present. We realise this could be upsetting if readers are looking for reassurance in the face of overwhelming upset, fear and chaotic thinking.

Third, it gives us all an opportunity to discover something new about human beings. We think it's best to be honest from the outset and say that we, along with all other mental health professionals, are still learning about human psychology. There are very few things that even the best experts are sure about. In a very real sense, this is upsetting to many of us. Whenever we are frightened or upset, it is perfectly natural to seek reassurance, and probably the first thing we look for are the answers to the questions, 'What is happening?' and 'Why is this happening?' What this book offers, in the face of uncertainty, is a way of thinking that is positive, hopeful and critical. We hope it is helpful too.

The nature of psychological distress

Feeling distressed and being different

It is often said that everyone is different. Yet being *too* different makes a person stick out in the crowd and this can be uncomfortable, to say the least. Being seen as 'different' is often the catalyst for bullying at school, attracts unwelcome attention as an adult and, depending on the 'difference', can even lead to a diagnosis of mental illness.

Taking just one example, until 1973, being gay was a diagnosable mental illness in the *Diagnostic and Statistical Manual of Mental Disorders*, the primary manual of psychiatric diagnoses used in the Western world and published by the American Psychiatric Association. Now that psychiatry has caught up with society, it is clear to us all that different sexualities are just that: differences between people, not an indication of illness.

Differences in sexuality are expressions of human individuality that should be accepted or celebrated, not diagnosed. When people are judged as bad or ill simply because they are different, the resulting stigmatisation can, in turn, make a person feel so distressed, ashamed and isolated that they experience symptoms that could be diagnosed as, for example, 'depression'. Studies show that a higher than usual number of gay men and lesbians attempt suicide, for example (Lee et al., 2017; Ryan et al., 2009).

This is a 'double whammy' that results from natural differences being judged negatively. Then, instead of explaining that such differences are simply expressions of human variation, medicine and psychiatry can make things worse by telling us that these experiences are illnesses; that there is something sick or defective about us.

It's also true that people's experiences of being different are also – well – different. That is to say, most people will be comfortable with being different in some respects, but not others. Everyone has different tolerance levels, but for most of us it is particularly difficult to endure being different in a way that attracts unwelcome attention in the form of bullying, discrimination, labelling and other stigmatisation. It is not 'character building'. So, if significant professional groups in society, the media and psychiatric diagnosis manuals say that the way that you are different is an unacceptable difference, it's likely that the experience of being different will be deeply unpleasant for you, simply because of the bullying, discrimination and stigmatisation that it attracts. Take away that unpleasant discrimination and differences have a much better chance of being accepted. We'll look at how stigmatisation and discrimination affect our happiness and mental health in Chapters 5 and 6.

Who is upset by distressing experiences?

Another problem with psychological distress is that it is sometimes as upsetting to witness it or have to deal with someone who is panicking, chaotic, agitated or overwhelmed, as it is to be suffering from any or all of these things. When we behave in a strange or disturbed way, we can be disturbing to those around us. Many, but not all, people who suffer extremely upsetting experiences are painfully aware that their behaviour has a disturbing effect on those around them, causing them further distress. As a result, they may keep themselves to themselves more, and this social isolation (a reasonable response to the world) is itself often seen as a diagnosable symptom of 'illness'.

If you are a witness to disturbing behaviour, you will most likely feel differently depending on whether the person in question is:

- a close friend or relative
- a life partner or spouse
- a passing member of the public
- the same or different ethnicity as you
- a man or a woman
- a child, adolescent or adult.

Each person has their own emotional reaction to disturbing behaviour and tries to make some rational sense of it according to their personal and professional perspective. Some of us will have a professional role, such as psychiatric nurse, social worker or police officer. Each response will, in some part, be determined by our beliefs about what causes psychological disturbance in general, and what has caused this distressing episode in particular. And each response will have the potential to help the distressed person or make them feel worse.

A key question is, 'How distressed is the person whose behaviour is so disturbing to me?' Not everyone who is disturbed is disturbing and not everyone who is disturbing is disturbed. It's not sensible to think that everyone behaving in a disturbing way should be diagnosed with a mental illness. What we experience as disturbing from moment to moment, situation to situation, is determined by many factors, including what we think is normal and the strength of our desire to live a quiet life, free from stress or threat.

All these complexities are conveniently brushed under the carpet by the illness model, or medical model, which argues that behaviour X is a symptom of illness Y. From this perspective, if you want to understand what is going on, the answer seems seductively simple: Y is causing X. This is not only far too simple; it can be dangerous. There is also a tendency in many societies to use the term 'mental illness' to identify and deal with people, behaviours and even ideas that are disturbing to the rest of us. We have already looked very briefly at how society included psychiatric diagnoses as a way of dealing with people who disturbed the comfortable norm in the case of sexuality. In their book *Making Us Crazy*, Kutchins and Kirk (1999) describe how the diagnosis 'masochistic personality disorder' was very nearly included in the third revised edition of the DSM, *DSM-III-R* (APA, 1987). Masochistic personality disorder was proposed (by a panel of psychiatrists) to be the tendency of people (mainly women) to provoke violence against them. So, a woman seeking sanctuary from domestic violence could have been diagnosed with a supposed 'mental illness' that caused her to invite violence towards her.

We will see throughout the book how ideas about what causes 'mental illness' are, at least in part, defined by the prevailing cultural beliefs in any particular society.

Psychological distress and illness

Western science, and most folk in the developed world, take the general view that mind and body are separate, which comes from a very long tradition of philosophy called dualism. Our present-day ideas were set out by French philosopher René Descartes in the 17th century. Believing that mind and body are separate lays the foundations for the idea that our minds are unaffected by events in our bodies, and vice versa. But we know from a mountain of scientific and personal evidence that, when something happens in our body, it can affect the way we think and feel (both positively and negatively, and to different degrees). We also know that some experiences affect the way our body works, such as anxiety (e.g. racing heart, feeling light-headed, breathlessness, tunnel vision). These links between mind and body then form chains – for example, being involved in a traumatic event will cause anxiety; anxiety can bring about very strong physical responses that themselves can be disturbing; this may lead to more anxiety. If this spiral of anxiety continues over a period of time, we might call it 'stress', which in turn triggers the release of a hormone, cortisol, which is intended to help us respond to whatever is causing the stress (fight or flight). However, if these high levels of cortisol persist over a long period, it can weaken the immune system, leading to numerous illnesses and, potentially, premature death. And so on… This is just one (highly simplified) example of the many interactions between mind and body that are a necessary part of life but can sometimes cause problems.

In short, we don't fully understand how our body and what we know as 'mind' actually bring about our experiences. This makes it genuinely difficult to separate the physical from the psychological, and this difficulty is important when we try to work out whether the physical and psychological events we find distressing are actually 'illnesses'.

When we feel overwhelmed by distressing feelings and chaotic thoughts, we can easily think we are suffering from an illness with a physical dimension. There can be real benefits in understanding experiences in this way:

- it gives access to a shared vocabulary – lots of people speak the

language of mental illness (not only doctors and other experts, but also, probably, some friends and relatives)
- it helps a person feel they are not the only one – they will not feel so isolated
- it gets access to treatments (both physical, such as medication, and psychological, such as talking therapies)
- it seems to offer a causal explanation for our distressing feelings.

However, many people, professionals and members of the public, do not think of these unpleasant experiences as an indication of illness at all, let alone as similar to a physical illness. Some think of the experiences as being simply different – possibly unusual and probably upsetting, but nevertheless only another expression of the range of human experience. The Hearing Voices Network, for example, regards hearing voices and other unusual experiences as normal variations of human experience and accepts each voice hearer's understanding of their voices without judgement.[1]

In this book, we invite you to consider how logical it is to think of distressing experiences as illnesses, rather than reasonable responses to an unreasonable environment.

When we say 'reasonable' response, we don't mean that all reasonable responses are necessarily immediately understandable to everyone. We think that the experiences and behaviour of people in distress are almost always meaningful to the person having them. We also think that understanding your own experiences better, and someone else understanding you too, is often the first step to feeling better. Finally, we challenge the evidence that they are caused by biological factors or chemical imbalances of the sort suggested in many textbooks and often in the media. You can make your mind up for yourself.

Our own experience as the basis of explanations

Many readers will know someone who has had a 'nervous breakdown' or suffers from a 'mental illness'. Many of you will have had experiences yourself that have been diagnosed as depression,

---

1. www.hearing-voices.org and www.intervoiceonline.org

anxiety, 'schizophrenia' and so forth. Others will only have come across the ideas in conversation or in the media. We have already suggested that your personal history will affect your ideas and, accepting that, we would like you to try to answer the following questions, based on your own experience. Is extreme human distress caused by:

- people being born with a faulty brain or nervous system?
- people being too sensitive and needing to toughen up emotionally in order to deal with today's world?
- a form of demonic possession?
- people being born with a tendency to respond in certain ways to stress, which will show itself if they have certain experiences, like bereavement, separation and divorce or childbirth?
- people growing up in chaotic, crazy families?
- people learning unhealthy ways of dealing with events in their lives that lead to upsetting symptoms when distressing events happen to them?
- a lack of spiritual strength or lack of disciplined faith?
- child abuse or neglect or other adverse events in childhood?
- something else?

We will look later at the evidence for many of these possible understandings. Some we can explain by looking at the history of ideas about the world; we can see that some understandings of madness are inextricably bound up with the zeitgeist, or 'spirit of the times'. It could be that some common understandings of madness turn out to be as realistic as believing that the earth is flat. In Chapter 2, therefore, we try to place ideas in their historical context. Whatever else history can teach us, we learn that our ideas are inevitably influenced by the views of most other people around us in whatever period we live, however accurate or silly those ideas are.

What you won't find in this book

Although this book is about the causes of mental health problems, we think that some readers will quite naturally want to link causes to treatments. If we know what causes distress, the next logical step is to turn our knowledge about causes into devising treatments to help people feel better. We have tried, however, to stick to our task, so readers will not find much about treatments in this book. For an honest evaluation of psychiatric treatments for mental health problems, we suggest readers take a look at Joanna Moncrieff's book on psychiatric drugs (Moncrieff, 2020) and Lucy Johnstone's book on psychiatric diagnosis (Johnstone, 2022), both in this same series.

We are also sure that people will devise their own theories about what may or may not help their friend, relative or themselves, based on their own exploration of possible causes.

Another thing you will not find in this book is a catalogue of categories of 'disorder', or lists of symptoms, with a further list of possible causes for each one. We don't have the space to include a comprehensive review of possible causes of each symptom or of each of the ever-increasing number of diagnostic categories to be found in the latest (fifth) edition of the *DSM* (APA, 2013) (or the 11th version of the *International Classification of Diseases*, the World Health Organization's equivalent diagnostic manual (WHO, 2019)). We realise that this, too, might be frustrating for readers who want answers quickly because they, their friends or their family are in extreme distress. There are two further reasons, apart from space, why we have not done this. First, it would almost certainly not be useful because, as we have hinted already, each list would be filled with unresolvable debates.

Second, we think that, given current disputes and debates, the best way of understanding an individual person's mental health problem is to understand that person, rather than their label or diagnosis (Boyle & Johnstone, 2020; Read & Moncrieff, 2022). All aspects of their life, past and present, are likely to hold clues as to why they are thinking and feeling the way they do. Nothing is automatically ruled out and, just as importantly, nothing is automatically ruled in.

We think this way of trying to understand mental health problems stands the best chance of locating real causal factors for each person. Furthermore, it lets us acknowledge that causal factors might well not be single events (an isolated biological malfunction or one-off experience of abuse) but might be sequences or accumulations of circumstances and events over time.

Chapter 2
A brief history of beliefs about the causes of human distress

Knowing the history of how people have thought about the causes of human distress, despair, madness and so on in previous centuries can be surprisingly helpful when trying to understand our own problems today. Others have done this in more detail (Cromby et al., 2013a; Foucault, 2006; Porter, 2002).[1]

First, history reminds us that there are many different ways to think about the causes. This can help us avoid getting stuck on just one, perhaps simplistic, explanation. Second, we can see that, although we do have more scientific approaches today than in the past, a big factor in determining which type of explanation dominates at any particular time and place is the world-view operating in that time and place. Furthermore, we can see that the dominant idea about how distress is caused can be useful to those with political or economic power. The flip side of that is that the theories (and the treatments justified by the theories) are often targeted at relatively powerless groups, such as women and poor people. People who simply don't fit in, who break contemporary social norms, can be described as mad, and causal theories are developed by 'experts' to prove that, and to explain why they need 'treatments' to be helped to become more 'normal'.

Last, we learn that there are three general types of causal theory that have been in competition with one another for centuries. These

---

1. This chapter is based on a previous book chapter by John Read (Read, 2013a).

three are nature, nurture and religion. The nature position argues either that people are born with problems or that the problems are caused by some malfunctioning in the body (often, but not always, the brain). The nurture (or environmental) position claims that we develop problems because of the bad things that happen to us, and/or by the absence of good things that should have happened but didn't. The religious position can involve punishment by the gods, but also sometimes involves the notion of people just being bad or immoral. Causal theories also vary as to the extent to which we hold the individual responsible for their own problems.

Gods and devils

Four thousand years ago, 'madness' was thought to result from the evil influence of some enemy, real or imagined. For example, the world view in Mesopotamia around 2000 BCE included the beliefs that evil demons were responsible for ailments and that the source of recovery was the appropriate good god. The demon responsible for madness was assisted by a collection of lesser demons and sorcerers, and the whole department was answerable to Ishtar, the female god supervising all witchcraft and evil (Alexander & Selesnick, 1996). The Persians and Hindus also believed evil gods – Ahriman and Shiva – were accountable for strange behaviours.

The earliest recorded attempts of the Hebrews to understand insanity also reflected the prevailing world-view (Miller, 1975; Rosen, 1964). Moses was clear about one cause: 'The Lord will smite thee with madness' (Deuteronomy, 28: 28). Moses also came close to providing an early example of this book's central theme – that madness is caused primarily by adverse life experiences: 'You shall be only oppressed and crushed continually; so that you shall be driven mad by the sight which your eyes shall see' (Deuteronomy, 28: 34). However, the ancient Hebrew theory remains one of divine punishment, since it is the Lord, rather than life events, that did the oppressing and crushing.

The world-view of the ancient Hebrews, in the Old Testament, included the notion that an efficient way to eradicate abnormal behaviour was to eliminate the person, rather than just the behaviour: 'A man or woman who is a medium or a wizard shall be put to death; they shall be stoned with stones, their blood shall be upon them' (Leviticus: 20: 27). The reason given by Moses for punishing a long list of behaviours by death was: 'So you shall purge the evil from Israel' (Deuteronomy 22: 22). Whether 'Israel' refers to a race or a country, this represents an early version of the primitive tendency to cleanse or eliminate unacceptable differences, which manifested centuries later in the eugenics movement (Read & Masson, 2013, 2022).

By the time of the first drafts of the Talmud (70–200 CE), the Hebrew world-view had changed. Now, before anyone could be punished for their behaviour, they must be considered responsible for it. While the Old Testament clearly held madness to be the direct result of sinning, the Talmud argued that the 'mad' were 'not responsible for the damage or the shame they produce', and they must, therefore, be helped rather than stoned or purged (Miller, 1975, p.529; Rosen, 1964, p.69).

The introduction of reason

Thinkers in Greece also indulged in magical and religious theories about unusual behaviour. Whether it was Ajax killing a flock of sheep believing it to be the enemy, or the daughters of Proteus believing they were cows and acting accordingly, there was a god to blame (Alexander & Selesnick, 1996, p.28).

There followed in Greece, however, what many describe as the most significant change in world-view that humanity has experienced. The 'Classical Era' was marked by the replacement of supernatural explanations with observation and reason. Priests were gradually replaced by physicians. The most famous doctor of all time, Hippocrates (460–377 BCE), was among the first to promote the 'medical model' of madness. He produced the first of many attempts to reduce the complexities of unusual, distressed or distressing human behaviours to a set of categories of illness, each with its own physiological cause:

> Men ought to know that from the brain and from the brain only arise our pleasures, joys, laughters and jests… Those who are mad through phlegm are quiet, and neither shout nor make a disturbance; those maddened through bile are noisy, evil-doers, and restless, always doing something inopportune. (Hippocrates, 1931, p.xvii)

As recently as 2022, a prominent British psychiatrist (Pariante, 2022) was still reciting the first sentence of this quote to refute a paper arguing that depression is primarily caused by depressing things happening (Read & Moncrieff, 2022).

Hippocrates was just as convinced as biological psychiatry is today that he really was discovering the physical causes of illnesses, rather than promoting a simplistic theory that conceals the complexities of unacceptable or disturbing behaviour and justifies and camouflages its social control. A sect called the Dogmatic school of medicine, or Dogmatists, was certainly convinced. Founded by Hippocrates' son and son-in-law in about 400 BCE, it was dedicated to prohibiting any investigation beyond the biological ideology of the day, because, they argued, Hippocrates had already discovered everything worth discovering. This attitude of certainty has been a feature of human thinking throughout history and remains so today in many areas of life. Any 'dogmatic' belief in a single system of explanation to the exclusion of any evidence to the contrary stymies discussion and sometimes renders reasonable debate impossible. While this book definitely leans toward psychological and social explanations of causes, we do not wish to prevent debate by proposing a fundamentalist psychosocial theory. Quite the contrary.

A chapter in *World History of Psychiatry* (Ducey & Simon, 1975) offers an insight, still valuable today, into one motivation for simplistic biological theories. The Greeks were becoming aware of human conflicts – not just internal conflicts regarding the motivations underpinning human behaviour, such as the 'reasoning' versus 'desiring' conflict identified by Plato (427–347 BCE) more than 2000 years before Freud, but also the conflict between the individual and the demands of society (see discussion of the 'id' versus the 'superego' in Chapter 7). In the absence of religious instructions regarding such dilemmas, there was a need to identify other forces over which the individual had little control and for which they could not be held accountable:

> The Hippocratic model of mental illness and of its treatment may have provided an important source of relief of anxiety, guilt and responsibility, by translating inner conflicts and

dissonances into physiological and physicalistic terms. (Ducey & Simon, 1975, p.19)

Hippocrates' treatments probably were effective in altering behaviour. Faced with being forced to vomit or defecate uncontrollably, or to swallow hellebore – a poison now used in insecticides – who wouldn't quieten down and agree that our behaviour was biologically based, especially if we knew that, if all that failed, blood-letting was the treatment of last resort?

During this period, there was a fading of an extreme male dominance that had included, for example, the feeding of boys at the expense of girls. When Plato wrote 'within the woman there is a wild, animalistic, Bicchantic [sic], frenzied creature, who must be gratified, or else she goes berserk' (Ducey & Simon, 1975, p.21), he wasn't suggesting that generations of oppression had led to pent-up anger, or that such oppression can drive women mad. He was laying the foundations for a quite different type of theory of female madness – a theory in keeping with the physiological explanations of the time and one that could be used not to liberate women but to continue their oppression.

The invention of 'hysteria' is an early example of the repeated, and continuing, use of biological theories of madness to force women into the roles determined for them by men.

Whenever the womb – which is an indwelling creature desirous of child-bearing – remains without fruits long beyond the due season, it is vexed and takes it ill; and by straying all ways through the body and blocking up the passages of the breath and preventing the respiration it casts the body into the uttermost distress, and causes, moreover, all kinds of maladies until the desires and love of the two sexes unite them. (Plato, 1904, p.916)

The treatments of choice for 'hysteria' were marriage and fumigation of the vagina. Although the experts told their 'patients' that the purpose of the 'treatment' was to attract the wandering uterus back to its rightful place, we can see with hindsight that it was the wandering of women from their subservient role that was the real concern.

A return to religion

The social structure of the mighty Roman Empire eventually crumbled before an onslaught of epidemics and marauding 'barbaric' tribes. The resulting insecurity led to a return to supernatural beliefs. By the 4th century CE, Emperor Constantine had made Christianity the official religion. The Church and State become an inseparable and immense power. In the field of madness, observation, reason and physiological theories were replaced with variations of the old religious themes. The Church became protector of the infirm and insane.

In the search for some external, and preferably heavenly, force to explain madness, it was thought that people tended to be particularly weird when alone at night – therefore, obviously, the moon was responsible for craziness. Mad people have, ever since, been called 'lunatics'.

Another concept, more consistent with Christianity, explained almost any anxiety-provoking event, including epidemics, conflagrations and madness, as witchcraft. This occasioned one of the most horrifying examples of the justification of violence by theories about groups of people considered different or defective. The targets of such violence are typically people, or groups of people, that best symbolise the nature of a society's collective anxiety. In this particular case, they were largely women.

The extent to which cultural changes influence theories about who or what is to blame for madness is well illustrated if we divide the Middle Ages (roughly the 5th–15th centuries) into two periods. In the earlier period, causal theories were influenced by the charitable aspects of Christianity. Care was relatively humane. Patients of the original Bethlehem Hospital in London, founded in the 13th century and variously known also as St Mary Bethlehem, Bethlem Hospital, and later the Bedlam 'snake-pit', wore arm badges when granted a pass out of the hospital. The response from the public was so positive that people who were not patients often counterfeited badges for themselves so that they would be treated equally favourably. (It was, perhaps, the equivalent of today's Blue Badge parking scheme.)

During this period, people accused of being possessed by the devil were not held personally responsible. The treatment, exorcism, was not a punitive process aimed at the individual but a benevolent one directed against the real cause of the problem – the Devil.

However, the breakdown of feudal structures that had occurred from the 11th century onwards, accompanied by insurrections that were often aimed at the Church, demanded scapegoats. Public trials and executions might deter other potential 'heretics'. But people seen to be possessed by the Devil could not be appropriate targets for punishment if they were not responsible for their actions. By the time Kraemer and Sprenger published their witch-hunting manual, *Malleus Maleficarum* (1486/1941), it had been 'discovered' that witches voluntarily invited the Devil into their lives. Thus, they were considered personally responsible for their 'possession', and the 'treatment' was to annihilate them.

Religious and social factors during this latter period of the Middle Ages had created an intense fear and hatred of women and a fiercely misogynist Church. *Malleus Maleficarum* described women as:

> a foe to friendship, an unescapable punishment, a necessary evil, a natural temptation, a desirable calamity… an evil of nature painted with fair colours. (Kraemer & Sprenger, 1486/1941, p.43)

Consequently, the vast majority of people tortured and murdered as witches were, indeed, women (Michelet, 1939). Many of them were guilty of nothing more than having healing skills, but their herbs and brews were seen as a threat to the male priests' monopoly on healing. Others were simply female and old. The symptoms are listed in the *Malleus Maleficarum*, the diagnostic manual of the day:

> All witchcraft comes from carnal lust which is in women insatiable… Three general vices appear to have special dominion over wicked women, namely, infidelity, ambition and lust. Therefore they are more than others inclined toward witchcraft who more than others are given to these vices. (Kraemer & Sprenger, 1486/1941, p.47)

The Inquisition, established by the Catholic Church initially in the 12th century to conduct trials of suspected heretics, is a horrifically clear example of a well-organised programme of cruelty directed against those engaging in behaviours considered unacceptable or inconvenient to those in power. Such programmes are often justified by theories disguising the violence as help for defective individuals. In the case of the women 'diagnosed' as witches, the 'help' took the form of being burned alive at the stake in order to 'purify' their souls so they could enter heaven.

The return to science

The return to observation and reason known as the Renaissance was a gradual process. For instance, Johann Weyer (1515–1561) used observation in his relentless battle against the idea of witchery. He demonstrated that objects that were alleged to have been implanted by the Devil in the stomach of an accused woman showed no signs of the effects of gastric juices. For this scientific discovery, he earned himself the diagnosis 'Weirus Insanus'.

An increased emphasis on the psychosocial origins of madness, or the 'nurture' position, were reflected in Shakespeare's *Hamlet* and Cervantes' *Don Quixote*. Burton's *Anatomy of Melancholy* (1621/1961), based partly on his need to understand his own chronic unhappiness, described one of the more popular diagnostic categories of this period. His theories were a blend of the demonological and physiological. Like those of his contemporaries, his treatments focused on exercise, diets, drugs and, typical of the era, purgatives. He added, however, a lovely description of one non-medical treatment for his own personal malady:

> It is the best thing in the world… to get a trusted friend, to whom we may freely and sincerely pour out our secrets; nothing so delighteth and pleaseth the mind, as when we have a prepared bosom, to which our secrets may descend, of whose conscience we are assured as our own, whose speech may ease our succourless estate, counsel relief, mirth expel our mourning, and whose very sight may be acceptable unto us. (Burton, 1621/1961, p.108–109)

Such a therapeutic experience was seldom enjoyed by thousands of Europeans who, under the guise of medical treatment, were being locked away, worked, purged and drugged. Soon after its opening in 1656, the Hôpital Général in Paris was 'treating' 6,000 people.

Typical of the view of this period taken by modern historians of psychiatry is the opinion that:

> The Age of Reason marked a great leap forward. Through the efforts of the great scientists, philosophers, men of letters, and artists of the 17th century mental illness was further extricated from superstition and authoritarian error. (Alexander & Selesnick, 1996, p.104)

However, on reflection, we think that the direction adopted during this period would turn out to be a transition from error based on one form of authority – religion – to error based on an equally dangerous form of authority – a particularly simplistic version, or perversion, of medical science.

Categorisation and confinement

From the latter part of the 17th century well into the 18th century, the 'scientific' approach to understanding the world established the dominance it maintains today. During this 'Enlightenment', explanations of madness became dominated by categorisation and physiology. Psychological and social factors were buried under the relentless drive to discover illnesses. However, the Enlightenment's many attempts to find the imagined true categories of 'mental illness' led to no useful advances in physiological explanations.

Herman Boerhaave (1668–1738), for instance, justified use of blood-letting and purgatives by his 'discovery' that 'melancholia' was caused by 'black juices'. His invention of the rotating chair was a particularly cruel form of so-called medical treatment that was explained by a variety of theories. For example, in Britain, Erasmus Darwin claimed that it reintroduced harmony to the 'disordered motions' of the nerves. Meanwhile, in North America, Benjamin Rush was telling patients that the reason they were being strapped to a board and spun into unconsciousness was to unclog their congested blood, which, he had discovered, was the true cause of madness.

The quest for specific brain pathology, still pursued today, was well under way. At London's Bethlem asylum, John Haslem was already conducting autopsies (Alexander & Selesnick, 1996, p.112). We might speculate as to how many of Haslem's subjects had died as a result of the poverty, neglect and violence that was endemic at the time. We might also note the enduring tendency to explain certain human behaviours using theories about disordered brains rather than the effects of social and economic conditions.

Who were these mad people? The 1656 Edict that founded the Hôpital Général defined its population as 'the poor of Paris, of both sexes, of all ages and from all localities, of whatever breeding and birth, in whatever state they may be, able-bodied or invalid, sick or convalescent, curable or incurable' (Foucault, 1967, p.39). The mad were locked away, not for being mad but for being poor.

The 'Great Confinement', as Michel Foucault describes this period (Foucault, 2006), served the economic function of forcing inmates to work at a fraction of the going rate, under the guise of exercise or 'occupational therapy'. While purporting to help the poor and sick, it served the political function of suppressing the increasing number of uprisings among the unemployed. It also bolstered a moral belief in hard work. The Edict deemed that the major causes of all disorders were begging and idleness – a theme that has tended to resurface in times of economic downturn and, most recently, so-called austerity (Friedli & Stearn, 2015).

Moral treatment

Philippe Pinel in France and William Tuke in England are remembered for their humane treatment of mad people. Their approach, a good example of the religious position on the causes of mental health problems, has come to be known as 'moral treatment' (Scull, 1981). Pinel, renowned for unchaining the insane, found it impossible to tell the difference between the effects of madness and the effects of cruel treatments in hospitals. Unlike many of the experts before them, Pinel and his fellow reformers were honest about being in the business of imposing society's moral code on deviant individuals. Pinel was particularly concerned to eradicate celibacy, promiscuity, apathy and laziness. Such a morality was a special goal for women because 'marriage constitutes for women a kind of preservative against the two sorts of insanity which are most inveterate and most often incurable' (Foucault, 1967, p.258).

Tuke founded the York Retreat in 1792, inspired by the values of his Quaker upbringing. His son, Samuel, who succeeded him, believed that 'to encourage the influence of religious principles over the mind of the insane is considered of great consequence as a means of cure' (Tuke, 1813, p.121). Patients were invited to tea parties with the staff and were expected to comport themselves with good manners.

But moral treatment had little impact on the stranglehold of biological theories about madness. The categorisations and the quest for physical explanations continued. For instance, despite producing an important treatise on psychotherapy in the early 19th century, Johann Reil lumped together all mute patients into a single category, for which he prescribed the treatment of standing next to cannon fire (Reil, 1803).

Aliens and alienists

The occasional critical voice could be heard. Jean-Pierre Falret (1794–1870) went beyond Pinel's questions about the effects of cruel treatment and wondered whether the language being used might be similarly damaging. He suggested replacing 'mental disease' with 'mental alienation'. He was drawing attention to the processes by which we can become disconnected from other people and from society as a whole. He renamed those trying to help people reconnect 'alienists'. The medical profession was unimpressed.

History in a nutshell

To summarise, there seem to be at least four themes, rules if you like, about how society tends to respond to 'madness':

1. 'Treatments' often seem to have the effect of suppressing behaviours, thoughts or feelings that are unacceptable to the majority or to those in power.
2. Those treatments have frequently been unhelpful and sometimes blatantly damaging.
3. There always seem to be experts who will argue that these ineffective or damaging treatments are actually for the good of the individual, who is seen as defective or abnormal in some way and in need of 'help'. These experts develop causal theories that justify the 'treatments' and locate the problem to

be solved firmly within the individual rather than in their life circumstances.

4. The way we think about people who are very distressed seems always to be contaminated by our tendency to want to separate 'them' from 'us' – to exaggerate the differences between the 'abnormal' and the 'normal', the 'mad' and the 'sane'. For centuries, this has involved locking them away somewhere out of sight, in places that symbolise our fear of insanity, of difference.

We hope we have shown that there has always been a range of explanations of madness competing for our attention. So, any debates you have been having with yourself, or others, about whether you were born with your problems or acquired them along the way (or a bit of both), and how responsible you, or your family, friends or others, are for causing them, have been going on for centuries. That may or may not be reassuring.

Chapter 3
The 20th century and beyond: the illness model

When a police officer asked a drunken man why he was peering at the ground around a lamp post, he said that he was looking for his keys. It was obvious that there were no keys on the pavement, so the officer asked why the man was looking for them under the streetlamp when he must have dropped them somewhere else. The man explained that he was looking under the streetlamp because the light was better there.

The age-old nature vs nurture debate continued into the 20th century. Up to the 1950s, the idea that psychological distress and disturbance were caused by 'nature' continued to be pursued by dedicated biological researchers supporting the theories of doctors and scientists whose interests lay in the 'medical model'. At the start of the 20th century, just about the only arguments for the 'nurture' side of the debate were those presented by Sigmund Freud's psychoanalytic theory.

However, the emerging field of social and behavioural science soon began to gain ground. Although at odds with Freud on the majority of points of philosophy and theory, the new science of behaviourism championed by John B. Watson and Frederick B. Skinner became the standard bearer for the nurture point of view. Human psychology – our personality, motives and behaviour, both how they developed and how they fell apart – was considered to be developed through interaction with the environment, rather than inborn. The behavioural science perspective on mental distress infused the mid-20th century with a new enthusiasm for looking for a cause of mental distress. Behaviourists' experiments (see Chapter 7) had shown that much of human behaviour is caused by 'reinforcement' (Watson & Rayner, 1920).[1]

On the nature side of the debate, treatment successes were claimed, in the 1930s and beyond, for both lobotomies and electroshock treatment, but subsequent scrutiny has raised serious questions about their effectiveness and safety (Read et al., 2019).

Meanwhile, psychiatry's genetic theories about unwanted behaviours had merged with the eugenics movement to lead, in the 1930s and 1940s, to the tragedy of the sterilisation of hundreds of thousands of people in America and Europe and the mass murder by the Nazi regime of about a quarter of a million psychiatric patients (Read & Masson, 2013, 2022). The fact that this did not lead to a reduction in 'mental illness' in the next generation is a strong indication that the genetic theories used to justify the sterilisations and killings were false.

In the early 1950s, the search for explanations for mental distress took a path that has dictated the discourse right up to the present day. The pharmaceutical industry and a psychotechnology dedicated to the medicalisation of all of life have generated an endless array of 'illnesses' and 'disorders', with an attendant array of new drugs to 'treat' them.

Our search for causes is inextricably intertwined with this development. We have to pause and ask, 'What is it that we are trying to understand the cause of?' We ask this now because, in a relatively few words since the beginning of Chapter 1, we have covered several thousand years of attempts to understand disturbance and distress. In that period, there have been times when the overarching explanations have changed ('religion', 'reason', and so on), but from the 20th century a new way of looking at human behaviour in general, including distress, began

---

[1]. See also the All About Psychology website (www.all-about-psychology.com) and the Classics in the History of Psychology website (www.yorku.ca/pclassic), including "'Superstition" in ther Pigeon', a fascinating journal article by B.F. Skinner (it's quite scientific): http://psychclassics.yorku.ca/Skinner/Pigeon

to dominate Western societies. In our attempt to understand the world, we have brought scientific methods to bear on our search for meaning. This is not necessarily a problem, unless it is applied with a peculiar twist: the tendency to see everything in medical terms so that all behaviour becomes medicalised.

In the 1970s, computerised axial tomography (CAT) and magnetic resonance imaging (MRI) scans helped scientists create visual representations of the human brain as it worked. These increasingly sophisticated techniques were pressed into service to look at the working brains of people diagnosed with different 'mental illnesses' to see if there was any difference in structure or function between them and the brains of 'normal' people.

The potential of these and other emerging neuroimaging techniques for revealing brain structure and function led to the then US President George Bush declaring the 1990s 'The Decade of the Brain', in order to 'enhance public awareness of the benefits to be derived from brain research'.[2] It was to be a public- and privately funded collaborative research initiative involving, among several institutions and agencies, the National Institutes of Health and the National Institute of Mental Health. In the search for causes, the spotlight was turned on brain structure and function via these exciting new technologies.

Another scientific innovation that influenced our search for causes was the Human Genome Project,[3] launched in 1990, which came to fruition with the publication of the complete human genome in 2003.

So the vast majority of research into the causes of mental health problems undertaken in the second half of the 20th century was into either genes or brains. A 2008 analysis, for instance, found that, for every study into the social causes of psychosis, there had been 15 into biological factors (Read et al., 2008). Many of the brain researchers seemed not to understand that brain differences between two groups of people (e.g., depressed and happy) revealed by neuroimaging techniques tell us absolutely nothing about the causes of mental health problems. This is because the brain has evolved specifically to interact with, and be changed by, the

---

2. www.loc.gov/loc/brain/proclaim.html

3. www.ornl.gov/sci/techresources/Human_Genome/home.shtml

environment. So, if you look at someone's brain after a loved one has died, it will indeed look different from the brain of someone who has just fallen in love (and it will look different too from the same brain at other times in the person's life). The essential question remains unanswered – which has caused the sadness: the bereavement or a collection of neurotransmitters? Indeed, not only is the question unanswered, but we maintain that it is unanswerable when asked from the poles of the nature–nurture debate. It is a complex system of interactions between events in the world and neurochemistry. There is, however, no need to have a 'chicken-and-egg' debate. In this instance, the sadness was clearly precipitated by an event in the world – the loss – which caused a cascade of internal responses, one of which was neural activity, all leading the person to feel 'down'. Furthermore, this is a natural, reasonable, indeed healthy response to an event in the world, not the result of some aberrant neurons. We must always remember to be very careful how we understand what is a 'healthy' and 'unhealthy' (normal/ abnormal, sane/insane) response in any given situation.

It has been shown that all the unusual features of the brains of people diagnosed with 'schizophrenia' (frequently described as a 'brain disease') are found in the brains of young children who have been severely traumatised (Read et al., 2001a, 2014a).

The drive to medicalise more and more behaviours led researchers to make claims about more and more 'illnesses' and 'disorders' – not only for 'mental illnesses' but for just about every facet of human life, from gambling to unemployment, from being overweight to criminality, from shyness to alcoholism. Many of the studies claiming to find the gene for this or that were later called into question or proved to be simply wrong, but by then we had read headlines like 'Schizophrenia Genes Identified', which is a far better story than 'Follow-Up Studies Fail to Reproduce Findings of Earlier Study'. In 2008, a paper in the *American Journal of Psychiatry* (Sanders et al., 2008), described by the editor as 'the most comprehensive genetic association study of genes previously reported to contribute to the susceptibility to schizophrenia' (i.e. a review of all previous studies), found 'nothing outside of what would be expected by chance' (Hamilton, 2008). There is, in fact, little evidence for a genetic component in most mental health problems, including depression and 'schizophrenia' (Hahn, 2019; Joseph, 2005, 2022a, 2022b; Ross, 2020).

The 'biopsychosocial' model

As early as the 1960s and early 1970s, there was some excellent research on the family's contribution to mental health problems and to the role of broader social factors like poverty (more about this in Chapter 6). A solution, or the appearance of a solution, to these two competing models – nature vs nurture, biology vs social factors – thence emerged.

In the 1970s, an integration of the two models was attempted. It became known as the 'biopsychosocial' approach, but was also sometimes called the 'stress-vulnerability' model. The idea was that we each have a varying degree of vulnerability to depression, anxiety, psychosis and so forth, and that this vulnerability is triggered by social stressors like poverty, neglect and violence. This model assumes, for example, that depressing events by themselves are not enough to make us very depressed – only those of us with a genetically inherited predisposition to get depressed or some other 'constitutional' vulnerability (maybe due to our mother's poor diet or smoking during pregnancy) will respond to those events with extreme depression. The greater your inherited or constitutional vulnerability, the smaller the amount of stress needed to tip you over the edge.

This sounds like a good idea, giving equal weight to biology and the social environment – nature and nurture. The problem, however, is that, because of the dominance of biological thinking, it is assumed that the vulnerability has to be inherited genetically. This reduces the role of social factors like child abuse, unemployment, loss, poor living conditions and so on to mere triggers of an underlying genetic or constitutional time bomb. Only people who have the supposed genetic predisposition become depressed, alcoholic or mad (Read et al., 2008). It implies that social factors by themselves cannot cause mental health problems.

This is both inaccurate and unhelpful, but it provides the illusion of an integration, and many researchers and mental health professionals still refer to this model without realising that the vulnerability side of the equation can itself be caused by bad things happening during childhood. For example, if you are abused or neglected as a child, you are more vulnerable to stresses (especially similar ones) later in life. Indeed, the inventors of the stress-vulnerability model (Zubin & Spring, 1977) clearly stated that there could be 'acquired vulnerability', which could be caused by 'the influence of trauma, specific diseases, perinatal complications, family experiences, adolescent peer interactions, and other life events that either enhance or inhibit the development of subsequent disorder'.

Although we are, of course, born with genetic variations (including, quite probably, differences in our general sensitivity to stress), you don't need a genetic predisposition for bad things to overwhelm you, make you depressed or drive you crazy.

Better solutions to the nature–nurture debate

So, we think the biopsychosocial or stress-vulnerability attempt to resolve the debate is only helpful if we acknowledge that the vulnerability side of the equation can be due to both our genetic make-up and/or the social environment we grow up in.

We now know, however, that just about everything we do, think or feel as human beings is partly determined by nature (our genes, brains and so forth) and partly by nurture (our upbringing, current circumstances and so forth). Some researchers have pointed out that it is, moreover, impossible ever to calculate what percentage of a given behaviour or problem, such as depression, is due to genetics and how much to the environment (Rose, 2005). They point out that genes have no influence whatsoever without an environment, and vice versa. They further remind us that, as soon as the first cell divides in the developing embryo, it has an environment. So where, they ask, does genetics end and the environment begin? They just cannot be separated in the way that many well-intentioned researchers have tried to do in the past. After reviewing the science, the eminent British clinical psychologist, Professor Richard Bentall, concluded:

> Finally, substantial resources have been spent, and continue to be spent, in the attempt to discover the genetic origins of mental illness, whereas its social origins continue to be

neglected... In this context it is important to note that no patient, not a single one, has ever benefited from genetic research into mental illness... Indeed, from the point of view of patients, there can be few other areas of medical research that have yielded such a dismal return for effort expended. (Bentall, 2009, pp. 144–145)

It seems that the whole genes vs environment debate, which has been going on for centuries, has been rather a waste of time. The two sets of factors are constantly interacting in an extremely complex way, such that is impossible to get a handle on it if simple answers are what you're after. To complicate matters further, recent discoveries in epigenetics (the study of how genes interact with their environment) have shown that the genes can be turned on and off by environmental factors (Champagne & Curley, 2009; Read et al., 2009). However, having the debate, even though it might seem sometimes overly academic and out of touch, has taught us just how complex really useful explanations are likely to be. Neither side of the debate should be dismissed if we truly want to understand the causes of psychological distress.

We think the best way forward is to stop trying to figure out whether 19% or 32% of depression or 'schizophrenia' is genetically determined and focus instead on determining the effect of factors that we can actually do something about. We don't think it's helpful to focus primarily on genetic factors, since recent history is laden with examples of how we have handled this idea poorly. We hope and expect that the vast majority of readers would agree that we don't want to return to the compulsory sterilisation programmes conducted in the USA, Scandinavia and Germany in the 1930s to try to eliminate the supposed genes from the gene pool (Read & Masson, 2013). But a version of this still occurs in the USA today in the guise of 'genetic counselling' to encourage some people not to have babies. If poverty, child abuse and such social ills are causes of something (with or without a genetic predisposition to that thing), then surely it is far more useful to focus on them and do something to prevent them (Clements & Davies, 2013).

This argument applies as much to the individual's efforts to understand the causes of their own problems as it does at a societal level. You might be reading this book because you want to understand the causes of your problems a little better, or maybe you want to learn about the causes of psychological disturbance in general. You might also be reading this book because you actually want to do something about those problems. Of course, having a new understanding can sometimes make a big difference all by itself – especially if someone has compounded their problems by blaming themselves or calling themselves 'ill', with the inevitable implication that they can do little or nothing to change.

But sometimes, for things to get better, we have to take our new understandings and actually use them to do something different. So, can you do anything about a person's genetic make-up? Can you do anything about the effects, in the present, of a lonely or scary childhood, about a stressful work situation, about a bullying family member, about being unemployed? What we are trying to say here is that spending time thinking, or worrying, about how much of a person's problem has been inherited is not going to get us very far. If we are looking at causes because we are really trying to find solutions, it is better to look at those factors that we are more likely to be able to influence.

The brain and biology

But what about the brain in all this? Of course our brains and our general biological make-up are important when it comes to understanding mental health problems. It's just that a disproportionate amount of attention has been paid to these factors by comparison with social causes, and any brain differences discovered have been wrongly assumed to be causal in nature (Cromby et al., 2013b).

A lot of information leaflets and websites, often funded by drug companies (De Wattignar & Read, 2009; Read & Cain, 2013), will tell you that you have an 'illness' that is caused by a chemical imbalance or some other 'brain abnormality'. For example, the American Psychiatric Association still promotes the ideas that 'Depression (major depressive disorder) is a common and serious medical illness' and that 'Schizophrenia is a chronic brain disorder'.[4] This is one of the common arguments of those who believe that brain differences show that nature is more important

---

4. https://www.psychiatry.org/patients-families

than nurture. But, as we have already seen above, the idea that brain differences imply an illness or disease does not necessarily hold up. What use would a brain be if it did not respond to what is happening around you? It is perfectly natural for your brain to be different when scary or depressive things are happening to us. It is another thing to say that those brain changes are the cause of our anxiety or depression.

Disease-centred versus drug-centred explanations

A disease-centred explanation

This argument – that complex, distressing experiences labelled as 'depression' or 'schizophrenia' and so on are illnesses caused by chemical imbalances in the brain – is often used by biologically oriented professionals in the mental health field, even though there is no robust evidence to support the argument (Moncrieff et al., 2022; Read, 2013b).

To justify this claim, they usually work backwards from the finding that the drugs used to try to mitigate the problem change certain chemical processes in the brain. The argument goes that, if drug X lessens some of the symptoms of the experiences labelled as 'depression', and we know that drug X increases the levels of chemical Y in the brain, then depression is caused by a deficit of chemical Y.

So, for example, it was noticed that paroxetine (trade names Seroxat, Paxil) affects pathways in the brain by increasing the level of the neurotransmitter serotonin. Taking paroxetine appears to reduce a range of symptoms associated with the diagnosis of 'depression'. Therefore, low levels of the neurotransmitter serotonin must, it was assumed, cause depression.

This is known as a disease-centred model because it hinges on the idea that a disease process causes the chemical imbalance that is subsequently relieved or restored by the drug. We will look at the evidence for this model later in this chapter. In her book *A Straight Talking Introduction to Psychiatric Drugs* (Moncrieff, 2020), British psychiatrist Joanna Moncrieff points out that the logic of the argument is similar to saying that, since we notice that drinking alcohol helps people overcome their inhibitions and become more socially outgoing, that proves that shyness (or 'social anxiety disorder') is caused by a lack of alcohol in the brain. Or that, because aspirin relieves headaches, headaches are caused by a lack of aspirin in the bloodstream. Moncrieff suggests, instead, a drug-centred model to explain the effects of psychoactive medications.

A drug-centred explanation

Note that, although we have used the example of paroxetine and depression, the models and their respective logic hold true for practically all diagnoses and psychoactive drugs. So, for example, the same relationship is posited between the symptoms of the experiences diagnosed as 'schizophrenia' and levels of the neurotransmitter dopamine and the drug chlorpromazine (Read, 2013b).

Moncrieff's drug-centred explanation would say that psychoactive drugs act by inducing a state of intoxication that might help the person taking the drug, make them feel worse, give them some relief from symptoms but with some unpleasant side effects, or have no noticeable effect. The drug-centred model is so called because it focuses on the drug and doesn't invent the notion that there is an illness that the drug is directly affecting, rebalancing or curing. In the drug-centred model, the relationship between the symptoms and the drug's action:

- might have some systematic elements (affecting all people in much the same way) by virtue of what we know about the physiology of the drug's effects, but
- will always have some idiosyncratic benefits or drawbacks as well (affecting individual people positively or negatively in unpredictable ways).

Using the same examples that we used in the section on disease-centred models, we can see that alcohol intoxication has the general side effect of taking away inhibitions, so the welcome effect on shyness and social anxiety is a specific action of the drug, but it does not mean that it cures shyness. Similarly, we know that aspirin has a general analgesic (painkilling) effect – in particular it helps toothache and headache. However, no one believes that aspirin cures headache or toothache by rebalancing chemicals in the brain or getting rid of infection in the teeth.

So a drug-centred model is accepted by many people as the real mechanism by which many drugs exert their beneficial effects. We are not alone in thinking that it is a better model for understanding drug action than proposing that psychoactive drugs are actually correcting imbalances in neurotransmitters or other chemicals in the brain.

The reason we have gone into some detail about treatment methods here is because theories about causes grow from retrospective observations about what works. Sometimes these are helpful and even turn out to be correct. Sometimes they are unhelpful and send searches for causes up cul-de-sacs while wasting valuable time and resources on the false trails.

Examples of theories of neurochemical malfunction

It is widely thought that brain chemicals called neurotransmitters contribute to the development of distressing experiences. In particular, the neurotransmitters serotonin and norepinephrine appear to play key roles.

As described above, originally, it was thought that low levels of these chemicals in the brain caused depression, but further research suggested that it is more complicated than that. More evidence encouraged some scientists to think that these two chemicals might regulate other neurotransmitters, such as dopamine and acetylcholine, that might also contribute to depression (Rampello et al., 2000; Janowsky & Risch, 1984). Later, the hormone melatonin was also thought to play a role in depression. In winter, the decrease in sunlight causes the human body to produce more melatonin, which results in greater fatigue and the need to sleep more (Wetterberg, 1999). Some people are affected more strongly by this production of melatonin, resulting in what is called seasonal affective disorder (SAD) (Dilsaver et al, 1990; Blehar & Rosenthal, 1989), leading to the idea that SAD is a form of depression.

This short excursion into a fragment of the research into neurotransmitters and 'mood' demonstrates that, when we delve into brain function to see what possible evidence there might be to involve neurotransmitters in symptoms associated with various psychiatric diagnoses, the situation is not at all clear. We pretty soon find out how little is actually known about how what we think might happen in the brain is translated into real world experience. Getting one person's experience to match a picture generated by a brain scan is difficult enough, but it then becomes clear that, to an important extent, everyone is different!

Nevertheless, it is possible to hypothesise what problems might be occurring. If we continue with the diagnosis of depression as our example, there could be:

- low levels of production of serotonin by brain cells
- a normal level of serotonin being made, but a lack of receptor sites able to receive the serotonin that is made
- a problem preventing serotonin from reaching the receptor sites
- a shortage of the chemical from which serotonin is made (this is known as a 'precursor' – in the case of serotonin a common substance called tryptophan, found in many foods).

If any of these neurochemical problems occur, theorists suggest it could lead to depression. In addition, theorists think that serotonin pathways might be implicated in obsessive-compulsive behaviour and anxiety. Indeed, anxiety is also widely seen as the key driver to many symptoms associated with mood problems, so this is not an unusual suggestion. However, it also demonstrates just how complex and interconnected the brain systems are – we can pretty soon come to the conclusion that serotonin is linked to everything and then the hypothesis loses any predictive power in relation to specific mental health problems.

Although it is widely believed that a lack of serotonin plays a role in depression, there are currently no techniques to measure serotonin levels in the living brain. It follows that there have not been any studies actually proving that brain levels of serotonin – or any other neurotransmitter for that matter – are in short supply when depression (or, indeed, any diagnosable mental illness) occurs (Moncrieff et al., 2022). However, blood levels of serotonin are measurable and there is some evidence to show that they are lower in people who suffer from depression (Hanh Le Quan-Bui et al., 1984). Among the several problems with such findings (including disputes about whether they can be repeated), we find that it still can't be shown whether the claimed low serotonin levels cause the symptoms of depression or the depression causes serotonin levels to drop.

So, both the evidence and the theories of neurochemical involvement in depression are, to say the least, incomplete (Moncrieff et al., 2022). They should be considered works in progress. It is really difficult to pin down straightforward relationships between neurochemical events and experiences.

Finally, you may have noticed that we slipped into the above paragraphs the fact that the precursor for serotonin is tryptophan. We did this so we could show how a very wide range of explanations and theories can spring up from rather scant and unreliable evidence. In the first place, it is an undisputed fact that tryptophan is the precursor to serotonin. Serotonin is effectively made from tryptophan. Tryptophan, however, is not manufactured in the body – it is an 'essential' amino acid – we have to eat foods that contain it. And this fact gives rise to theories that experiences likely to be diagnosed as depression can be affected by the amount of tryptophan in the diet. In simple terms: eat more tryptophan and you'll cheer up (see, for example, Jenkins et al., 2016). Indeed, a quick internet search turns up a lively debate about a suggestion that it's the tryptophan in turkey that causes Americans to feel so benign at Thanksgiving.

There are, of course, many explanations for why someone might have a feeling of wellbeing after eating turkey that are a lot more plausible than the amount of tryptophan it contains! It turns out that tofu, cod, cheese and pork all contain more tryptophan than turkey. We can see, though, how human imagination, set free from the discipline of scientific evidence, can come up with explanations that have superficial plausibility.

The jury remains out, not only on the mood-lifting properties of tofu and turkey but also on the particular role of serotonin in depression. In 2022 an international group of psychiatrists analysed 17 previous reviews of serotonin-depression research studies. They found 'no consistent evidence of there being an association between serotonin and depression, and no support for the hypothesis that depression is caused by lowered serotonin activity or concentrations' (Moncrieff et al., 2022).

Can drugs cause psychosis?

It has been known for thousands of years that certain substances have a mood-altering effect. More recently we have discovered a little about how this happens. Morphine, cocaine, alcohol, caffeine, cannabis and psilocybin (found in 'magic mushrooms') are just a few of the better known of these substances. Most readers will have taken one or more of them and experienced their effects. These effects are caused by their action on our neurotransmitter systems. Some substances (e.g. alcohol) have an effect on many neurotransmitter systems at once, and these effects can work in complex ways, sometimes against each other:

- alcohol affects the dopamine system, making you feel excited
- alcohol affects the glutamate system, causing muscle relaxation and slurred speech
- alcohol affects the gamma-aminobutyric acid system, making you calm and drowsy.

Other substances (e.g. morphine and cocaine) have a very discrete effect on one system only and have been called 'chemical scalpels' because they are so specific in their action that they can be used with precision in medical treatments.

When it comes to understanding distressing psychological symptoms, there is an inescapable logic in the idea that, if some drugs appear to lessen distressing symptoms, then other drugs might exacerbate them, or even be able to cause them in the first place. It is also possible that some substances might throw neurotransmitter systems out of kilter, temporarily or permanently. Add to that the fact that the effects of using substances like cannabis and magic mushrooms are experienced as being very similar to some of the symptoms of psychoses, and it's easy to hypothesise possible links.

In statistical terms there is a demonstrably reliable relationship between cannabis use and psychosis, but this is not completely straightforward. Some readers will have personal experiences of, or know others who have had, extremely unpleasant experiences after using cannabis. We know that cannabis is widely used in the Western world, particularly by adolescents – a time in people's lives that is particularly associated with the development of symptoms associated with a diagnosis of psychosis (Harrop & Trower, 2001). We also know that there is an association between cannabis use and the development of psychosis (Hall & Degenhardt, 2000). It's important to understand that an association between two things simply means that the two events are likely to occur together. It doesn't mean that one event causes the other. There are at least three logical possibilities in the case of cannabis and psychosis:

- cannabis use causes psychosis (variations on this idea are explored next)
- psychosis causes cannabis use (not as daft as it might seem, since we know that people will try all sorts of things to get rid of their symptoms, and alcohol and cannabis are high up on the list because some people find their effects calming or numbing)
- a third, unknown variable is causing this association. (An everyday example of this is the association between eating ice cream and drowning. Why is this? Because, when the weather warms up, more people go swimming in the sea and we eat more ice cream. But no one suggests that eating ice cream causes you to drown.) It's worth remembering this type of 'association' because it's usually the kind of finding that lies behind news headlines 'linking' 'schizophrenia' or other mental health problems with just about everything.

The active ingredient in cannabis is tetrahydrocannabinol (THC), which attaches itself to the cannabinoid receptors (found in three areas of the brain), and in research terms there are several possible hypotheses that might explain the link between cannabis use and symptoms. These are, in short form:

- cannabis causes psychosis
- cannabis precipitates psychosis in people who are predisposed to it
- cannabis causes changes in the brain that make us more likely to respond to stress with symptoms of psychosis
- cannabis makes symptoms worse in people who are already

suffering from unpleasant experiences and try to alleviate them by using cannabis
- cannabis causes temporary psychosis-like symptoms
- cannabis does not cause psychosis.

If we look at a wide range of research, it's difficult to come to a firm conclusion on whether or not cannabis use causes symptoms associated with psychosis. One study tried to separate out the effects attributable to cannabis and to childhood sexual abuse on the rate of psychosis (Shevlin et al., 2009). Readers will now appreciate some of the difficulties of working this out. Mark Shevlin and his colleagues looked at the development of symptoms in groups of people who had:

1. no sexual trauma or cannabis use (this is the reference group with which the other groups were compared – it gives a type of background level of diagnosis of psychosis)
2. sexual trauma with no cannabis use ever
3. cannabis use with no sexual trauma ever
4. first sexual trauma occurring before first cannabis use
5. first cannabis use occurring before first sexual trauma.

They found that, in comparison with group 1, group 2 were about twice as likely to receive a diagnosis of psychosis, whereas group 3 were no more likely to receive a diagnosis of psychosis than group 1. Group 4 were four times more likely to receive a diagnosis than group 1, and just about the same result was obtained for group 5. This was a complicated study that made adjustments for a number of factors.

From this study it looks as though on its own, cannabis use isn't a significant factor in the development of psychosis. Childhood sexual abuse, however, *is* linked to the development of psychosis, and when combined with cannabis use, it seems to become a really strong factor. This seems to support our general theme in this book – namely, that distressing experiences and symptoms that might be diagnosed as psychosis have many complex causes, including physical (biological/neurochemical), psychological (e.g. trauma or abuse) and social (e.g. poverty, unemployment).

In summary, drugs are consumed by people because they have an effect, but it's difficult to predict what distressing effects there might be from person to person. Trauma at any time of life can result in distressing reactions, and trauma during childhood is particularly likely to lead to adult symptoms and diagnoses of psychosis. Combining the two (whether or not the drugs are used as self-medication for the effects of trauma and so on) seems particularly potent, and we should therefore be arranging child protection, education and family support to take account of this.

Our conclusion is that, whether we focus on genes or the brain, the nature–nurture argument is not very helpful in understanding the causes of our problems and virtually useless when it comes to figuring out what we can do about those problems.

The remaining questions are: why do we as a society, and as a mental health culture established by professionals, seem to prefer to base our understanding on such a polarised debate? And why is there such a bias towards the view that nature is far more important than nurture in causing our problems? Biologically oriented mental health professionals – mostly but not exclusively psychiatrists – promote this view for several possible reasons, ranging from the understandable difficulty that some of them have to engage on a human level with very distressed or distressing people (preferring instead to keep their distance by just making a diagnosis and prescribing a drug), to a genuine belief that an illness explanation is more helpful because it avoids having to 'blame' anyone (see Chapter 5).

The pharmaceutical industry

Another influential group promotes illness explanations for more obvious reasons. No discussion of what happened to our thinking about the causes of mental health problems in the second half of the 20th century and beyond would be complete without looking at the role of the pharmaceutical industry. Most discussions ignore it completely. This is because, generally speaking, mental health researchers and professionals believe they are immune to economic and political pressures; they believe they are objective, scientific. We explained in Chapter 1 how we think it is practically impossible to be objective. We don't make this claim ourselves. We do, however, demand, and suggest everyone demands, transparency when it comes to vested interests in different types of explanation.

One of us (JR) was once asked to write an article for a new journal in the psychosis field (Read et al., 2008). To encourage him to accept the invitation he was told that the journal was sent free to 20,000 psychiatrists in the USA. He asked how those 20,000 were selected and was told that the drug companies provided the journal with a list of the 20,000 psychiatrists who had prescribed the most antipsychotic drugs in the preceding year.

Regardless of your position on the causes of mental health problems, most people now understand that the pharmaceutical industry has massive influence over mental health research, research journals, teaching institutions, professional organisations, drug-regulating authorities, the information we are offered over the internet, and even (especially in the USA) the politicians and bureaucrats responsible for our mental health services. After decades of silence, more and more professionals who are concerned by this situation are beginning to speak out (see, for example, Davies, 2013, 2021; Moncrieff, 2020; Sharfstein, 2005; Shooter, 2005). The final chapter of this book, updating this second edition, will report how the United Nations and the World Health Organization have recently joined in.

One problem is that many researchers, research programmes, journals, university departments and special interest groups have become dependent on drug company money (Healy & Thase, 2003; Mosher et al., 2013; Moynihan & Cassels, 2005). The industry has particularly expanded its influence by funding the websites of community groups. Studies show that about half of all websites set up by user/consumer/patient groups in the mental health arena are funded by the industry and that these sites are biased in favour of biological approaches to understanding and treating these conditions (Cosgrove & Krimsky, 2012; De Wattignar & Read, 2009; Read & Cain, 2013). When the fifth edition of the DSM came out (APA, 2013), 67% of the panel responsible for writing the sections on mood disorders and 83% of those coming up with the diagnoses for psychotic disorders had financial ties to drug companies (Cosgrove & Krimsky, 2012). This was actually an improvement on DSM-IV (APA, 2000, when *all* members of both panels had links with the industry.

The pharmaceutical industry is enormously wealthy and enormously powerful, conducting more and better research on how to market their products effectively than psychologists do on evaluating psychological treatments or service providers do on evaluating medication- free mental health services.

This single-track approach means that fewer and fewer people are able to actively seek explanations for distress outside of a very narrow band of possibilities. It is difficult to obtain funding or approval for research into psychological and social explanations when our day-to-day understanding is flooded with medical metaphors for distress and just about every problem in living, however minor.

A new century

There are, of course, many exceptions to simplistic, illness approaches. Throughout the world during the last century, many mental health professionals continued to try to work on a human rather than a chemical level. Will the 21st century see more support for psychological explanations? Will the social causes of mental health problems finally be given the attention they deserve?

The situation was summarised when, in 2005, the President of the American Psychiatric Association, Dr Steven Sharfstein, wrote:

> We must examine the fact that as a profession, we have allowed the bio-psycho-social model to become the bio-bio-bio model ... If we are seen as mere pill pushers and employees of the pharmaceutical industry, our credibility as a profession is compromised. (Sharfstein, 2005, p.82)

Professor Mike Shooter, President of the Royal College of Psychiatrists in the UK, added:

> I cannot be the only person to be sickened by the sight of parties of psychiatrists standing at the airport desk with so many perks about them that they might as well have the name of the company tattooed across their foreheads. (Shooter, 2005, p.31)

The ever-increasing prescription rates for psychiatric drugs, especially for children and the elderly, do not give cause for optimism. Let us take antidepressants as an example.

In 2000, 22 million prescriptions for antidepressants were given out in the UK. By 2007 this had surged to 34 million.[5] In 2017/18, 7.3 million adults (17% of adults) were prescribed antidepressants in one year in England alone, with higher rates for women, older people and people in deprived areas (Taylor et al., 2019). Prescribing continued to increase at roughly the same rate during the Covid-19 pandemic, with 20.5 million antidepressant drugs prescribed in England between October and December 2020, a 6% increase compared with the same quarter in 2019/20 (Taylor et al., 2019). Currently 2.1 billion doses of antidepressants are prescribed annually by GPs to a population of 52 million people in England (Heald et al., 2020). Similarly high prescription rates are found in Australia, Belgium, Canada, Iceland, Portugal and Sweden (OECD, 2021).

In America, in 2005, 5% of men and 11.11% of women in the USA were taking antidepressants (Moncrieff, 2020). By 2015–2018, this had risen to 8.4% of American men and 17.7% of American women, spiking at 24.3% among women aged 60 and older (Brody & Gu, 2020).

However, there are some signs that psychosocial explanations have not disappeared altogether. If we look at the diagnosis of 'schizophrenia', since the 1990s many studies have shown that factors like poverty, urban living, child abuse and other indicators of deprivation, destitution and violence are highly predictive of who ends up hearing voices or having delusions, with or without a genetic predisposition (Larkin & Morrison, 2006; Read et al., 2008; Moskowitz et al., 2019; Read, 2020; Varese et al., 2012).

An increasing number of psychiatric journals now have strict requirements about researchers declaring any funding from drug companies and other conflicts of interest. One recently launched journal, *Psychosis: Psychological, Social and Integrative Approaches*, the journal of the International Society for the Psychological and Social Approaches to Psychosis and other Psychoses, refuses

---

5. Statistics from the Health and Social Care Information Centre: www.gov.uk/government/organisations/health-and-social-care-information-centre

to take drug company advertising (its editor is John Read). Some governments and professional organisations have begun imposing restrictions on how much money psychiatrists (and other doctors) can receive from drug companies. The Norwegian Medical Association barred conference organisers from accepting drug company money if they want the conference to qualify as being 'educational'. Legislation now forces drug companies to disclose all of their studies, not just the few they select to submit to drug regulation agencies (which, naturally, tended to be those that came up with the most favourable results). This has at last led to comprehensive, rather than highly selective reviews of the research. One of these, for example, showed that antidepressants are, for the vast majority of recipients, no more effective than placebos (dummy pills) (Kirsch et al., 2008).

We finish with some warnings from neuroscientist Steven Rose, who powerfully outlines the dangers of looking for causes exclusively in an individual's biology:

> Consider the world-wide epidemic of depression identified by the World Health Organisation (WHO) as the major health hazard of this century, in the moderation – though scarcely cure – of which vast tonnages of psychotropic drugs are manufactured and consumed each year. Prozac is the best known ... Questions of why this dramatic rise in the diagnosis of depression is occurring are rarely asked – perhaps for fear it should reveal a malaise not in the individual but in the social and psychic order. Instead, the emphasis is overwhelmingly on what is going on within a person's brain and body. (Rose, 2005, pp.5–6).

He continues:

> The neurogenetic-industrial complex thus becomes ever more powerful. Undeterred by the way that molecular biologists... are beginning to row back from genetic determinist claims... psychometricians... behaviour geneticists... and evolutionary psychologists are claiming genetic roots to areas of human belief, intentions and actions long assumed to lie outside biological explanation. Not merely such long-runners as intelligence,

addiction and aggression, but even political tendency, religiosity and the likelihood of mid-life divorce are being removed from the province of social and/or personal psychological explanation into the province of biology. With such removal comes the offer to treat, to manipulate, to control. (Rose, 2005, pp.6–7).

It will require all of us, users of mental health services and mental health staff, to work together to create sufficient conceptual space and financial resources to bring balance to the important task of seeking explanations for madness.

Then, together, we can turn our 21st-century mental health services into ones where the first questions asked are not necessarily 'What are your symptoms?', 'What is your diagnosis?' and 'Are you taking your medication?', but 'What is troubling you?', 'What do you think has happened to bring this about?' and 'What do you need from us?'

Chapter 4
Do diagnoses help us understand causes?

In this chapter we explore the reasons why some people find diagnoses helpful, at least in the short term, and argue that they actually tell us little or nothing about the causes of or solutions to our problems, and can sometimes conceal the real causes and can even contribute to stigma and pessimism. The issues discussed in this chapter are dealt with in more depth and detail in another book in this series, *A Straight Talking Introduction to Psychiatric Diagnoses*, by British psychologist Dr Lucy Johnstone (2022).

When someone comes into contact with mental health services, they will probably (but not always) be given a diagnosis of some sort. Many of us even try to diagnose ourselves (or our loved ones), often by surfing the internet. Having a label to apply to our problems can be experienced as very helpful. At least we now have a word for what is happening to us (or, in medical terms, what illness we've got). It can sometimes also appear to give us an explanation. If there is a word that 'experts' use to describe our difficulties, then that suggests two things. First, other people must have the same problems, and that can be very comforting. Second, we might assume that the experts who have come up with the name for what's troubling us must know something about what causes it and how to 'treat' it. That is also reassuring. The last thing anyone wants to hear from their doctor is, 'Oh dear. I've no idea what's wrong with you.'

Psychiatric diagnoses, however, are something of a mixed blessing. As well as looking at the pros and cons of diagnoses we will briefly outline the nature and history of diagnosing and describe how it works in practice today.

Human beings can't help categorising and labelling

The human ability to categorise and label things in our world is extremely helpful. It is 'natural' to us – one of the first thought processes we develop as human beings. It is completely understandable, therefore, that humans have always applied labels to distressing or unusual behaviour. In Chapter 2, for example, we came across 'hysterics', 'lunatics' and 'witches'. A comprehensive history would produce hundreds of terms, tried and discarded over the centuries – and that's just in one culture. The task facing us, and our predecessors, has always been the same: to lump together a set of behaviours and apply a name to it, in the hope that somehow this will increase our understanding of what it is, what causes it and what to do about it.

There is a tradition in literature and the history of human ideas that suggests that, when we can name something, it gives us power over it. So, if we can name the disturbance or distress, we can categorise it and control it. This usually means putting it in a group with something that it appears to resemble and creating the illusion of a dividing line, in this case between the 'mad' and the 'normal' or between different types of 'mad'. The labels, which often sound a bit medical, a bit scientific, or at least a bit 'Latinish' – like 'melancholia' or 'dementia paranoides' – have sadly proved more effective at dividing 'us' from 'them' than increasing our understanding of what causes the problem in question.

Categorising and naming are essential for learning anything about the world, for storing the millions of bits of information that bombard us every day. Without being able to categorise, and thereby quickly recognise situations and people that are dangerous, we would not survive the first few years of life. So humans who *have* survived have become very good at categorising.

What do psychiatric labels tell us?

There are at least two problems, however, when we apply this skill to one another. First, since our survival sometimes depends on rapid categorisation, we all too quickly put people (including ourselves) in boxes. The labels on these boxes tend to stick around for a long time. Then we find we have put people into boxes from which they (we) can never escape. From that moment on, we interpret everything they do through the filter of our understanding that they are an 'x' sort of person. Second, we tell ourselves that we now understand why a person does what they do, why they are who they are and so on: 'Of course they act like "y" because they are a "y" sort of a person.'

Or, in the case of psychiatric diagnoses, 'Of course they do "schizophrenic" things – they are "schizophrenic".' It is worth remembering that this whole construction of assumed 'understanding' has come about simply because we have arbitrarily given something a label, and there is a huge difference between naming something and understanding it.

The important point here is that a diagnosis tells us nothing at all about what causes someone to act in a certain way. It is nothing more or less than an arbitrary label applied to a group of behaviours (or ways of thinking or feeling). This means that the reassurance gained from receiving a diagnosis, the belief that 'At least now I know what I've got and why I feel/act the way I do', is an illusion. All you really know is that a diagnosis is the word that experts use to label your behaviours, thoughts or feelings. They haven't understood it any better at all.

Although psychiatric diagnoses tell us nothing about the causes of mental health problems, it is notable that medical language (which tends to give it authority, even though there is still no understanding) is built into the 947-page *DSM-5*, the book most commonly used around the world to help mental health professionals decide what diagnosis to apply (APA, 2013). Almost every diagnosis (itself a medical-sounding word) ends with 'disorder'. For example, there's 'anxiety disorder', 'depressive disorder', 'panic disorder', 'intermittent explosive disorder' and 10 types of 'personality disorder' ('antisocial', 'narcissistic', borderline', 'avoidant' and so on). For our children, there's 'conduct disorder', 'oppositional defiant disorder', 'attention deficit hyperactivity disorder', 'communication disorder' and so on). In this way, our problems are made to sound like illnesses whether they are or not. Indeed, the behaviours, thoughts and feelings used to decide which 'disorders' we have are even called 'symptoms'.

The *DSM* itself acknowledges that it is 'atheoretical' and that it says nothing at all about causes. Nevertheless, its medical language implies that what are being described are illnesses. This choice of language, consistent with the overarching term 'mental illness', is unsurprising, given that the *DSM* is written by medical doctors (psychiatrists) from the country with one of the most biological approaches to mental health in the world, the USA, and most of these doctors have financial ties with drug companies.

It hasn't always been so. In the very first, much shorter, 1952 edition of the *DSM*, the same problems now called 'disorders' were all called 'reactions'. This was a different era, one in which psychoanalytic psychiatrists were in the ascendancy in the USA. Like the general public (see Chapter 5), they understood that mental health problems stem largely from life events and our interpretations of those events, rather than from faulty genes or imbalanced brain chemicals. The difference between believing that your difficulties are caused by your having some kind of biological disorder and believing that you are having an understandable, albeit upsetting, reaction to your life history and circumstances is enormous (Cromby et al., 2013c).

Medicalising distress can hide the real causes

This diagnostic approach to human distress medicalises all sorts of things, turning our reactions to life events into disorders. Feeling very sad after something sad has happened becomes major depressive disorder; being very nervous in lots of situations without really knowing why becomes generalised anxiety disorder. More and more problems have been redefined as 'disorders' or 'illnesses', supposedly caused by genetic predispositions and biochemical imbalances, with life events relegated to mere triggers of an underlying biological time bomb.

Excessive gambling, drinking, drug use or eating are illnesses. So are eating and sleeping too little and not having enough sex. Being painfully shy has become 'avoidant personality disorder'. Beating people up is now 'intermittent explosive disorder'. There are now so many disorders in *DSM*'s 947 pages that if you can't find yourself at least three times you probably have 'need to get a life disorder'.

Our children are labelled too. Being bad at sums has become 'mathematics disorder'. Ignoring other people's feelings (once called being naughty) means your child is suffering from 'conduct disorder'. If this also includes getting angry with grown-ups, the diagnosis changes to 'oppositional defiant disorder'. A diagnosis often in the news (because of alarming increases in the prescribing of amphetamines) is 'attention deficit hyperactivity disorder'. The 'symptoms' of ADHD include fidgeting, losing things, talking excessively and difficulty playing quietly or taking turns (APA, 2013, pp.59–60). Of course, children sometimes have problems. But does labelling them help in any way? Readers wanting to pursue this theme might be interested to read British child psychiatrist Sami Timimi's book in this series, *A Straight Talking Introduction to Children's Mental Health Problems* (Timimi, 2021).

Since the current book is about the causes of mental health problems, we ask whether diagnostic labelling of behaviours (however distressing to self or others they may be) actually takes us any nearer to understanding the cause of the behaviours. We think the answer is quite simply 'no'.

Furthermore, we are concerned that such labelling sometimes conceals the actual causes by locating the problem entirely within the individual adult or child. From such a viewpoint, there appears to be no value in prevention programmes to reduce things like abuse and neglect. We just need to medicate the 'sick' child.

This locating of the problem entirely in the individual is just one of the many downsides of a diagnostic/labelling/categorising approach to assessing mental health problems. A diagnostic approach also graces someone's arbitrary idea with a baseless 'scientific' authority. By giving the impression that something is actually known about this behaviour, a diagnosis also means that we stop looking for real explanations in the real world. The diagnosis itself, however arbitrary, substitutes for real explanation and understanding.

Are psychiatric diagnoses scientific?

There are two important if rather 'academic' issues to be considered here: reliability and validity. Reliability is the extent to which we can agree on what is in front of us: in this case, the extent to which experts agree on the diagnosis of the same person. Thirty-five years ago researchers found that, when 134 US and 194 British psychiatrists were given a description of a patient, 69% of the US psychiatrists diagnosed 'schizophrenia' but only 2% of the British psychiatrists did so. The majority of the British psychiatrists (75%) said the person had a 'personality disorder' – a view held by just 7% of their USA colleagues (Copeland et al., 1971). By 1992, researchers had identified 16 systems of classifying 'schizophrenia'. Out of 248 patients, the number diagnosed as 'schizophrenic' by these systems ranged from one to 203 (Herron et al., 1992).

The absurdity of all this was illustrated by a famous study in which 'normal' people were admitted to psychiatric hospitals complaining that they heard the words 'empty' or 'thud', and were all diagnosed 'schizophrenic'. None of the staff, but many of the patients, recognised that the 'pseudo-patients' were 'normal'. A follow-up study, in which hospital staff were told that 'pseudo-patients' would be admitted, produced a 21% detection rate by staff. But no 'pseudo-patients' had been admitted (Rosenhan, 1975)! American psychologist Lauren Slater considers this study one of the 'great psychological experiments of the 20th century' and conducted a small repeat version of it – with similar results (Slater, 2004). (Although, it should be noted that the accuracy of Rosenthal's original experiment has recently been questioned (Cahalan, 2019).)

Validity in research is when a construct is related to, or predicts, the things it is supposed to be related to or predict. Psychiatric diagnoses have, for instance, very little 'predictive validity' because they tell us so little about long-term outcomes. The British clinical psychologist Richard Bentall has this to say about the validity of psychiatric diagnoses:

> A wide range of evidence suggests that our current system of diagnostic classification has led psychiatry down a path that is no more scientific than astrology. Like star signs, psychiatric diagnoses are widely believed to tell us something specific about ourselves, to explain our behaviour and personality, and to predict what will happen to us in the future. Like star signs, diagnoses fail on all of these counts. (Bentall, 2004, p.195)

He continues:

Even if the reliability problem were one day solved, there would be no guarantee that the resulting diagnoses would be scientifically valid or clinically useful. If a disease is operationally defined in terms of an arbitrary but unrelated set of criteria a meaningless diagnosis can be assigned to patients with a high degree of reliability. This would be the case if, for example, we defined 'Bentall's Disease' in terms of such easily defined symptoms as hair colour, the number of summer colds experienced in the last five years, and the number of Pink Floyd albums owned. (Bentall, 2004, p.196)

Advantages and disadvantages of the diagnostic approach to understanding mental health problems

Advantages
- Assists communication (about research and treatment)
- Brings relief (through appearance of an explanation, and awareness that others have the same problem)
- Assists managers/policy makers to decide whose problems are serious enough to deserve treatment/funding

Disadvantages
- Tells us nothing about causes
- Locates problem entirely in individual
- Suggests an illness – ignores social causes
- Underestimates capacity for change
- Reduces hope of recovery
- Stigma and prejudice from diagnostic labelling
- Categories vs dimensions ('pigeon-holing' vs acknowledging that most of us have the problem to varying degrees at different times)
- Poor reliability (experts can't agree about who has got what)
- Poor validity (diagnoses don't predict future or our response to different treatments)
- 'Co-morbidity' (most of us have two, three, four or more *DSM* 'disorders')

In 2013 the British Psychological Society had this to say:

> It is timely and appropriate to affirm publicly that the current classification system as outlined in DSM and ICD, in respect of the functional psychiatric diagnoses, has significant conceptual and empirical limitations. Consequently, there is a need for a paradigm shift in relation to the experiences that these diagnoses refer to, towards a conceptual system not based on a 'disease' model. (BPS, 2013)

A year earlier, Dr Allen Frances, the Chair of the panel of eminent US psychiatrists that produced *DSM-IV*, wrote this of the fifth edition (*DSM-5*), which had just been published:

> This is the saddest moment in my 45-year career. The APA has given its final approval to a deeply flawed *DSM-5* containing many changes that seem clearly unsafe and scientifically unsound. My best advice to clinicians – be sceptical and don't follow *DSM-5* blindly down a road likely to lead to massive over-diagnosis and harmful over-medication. (Frances, 2012)

Stigma and prejudice

The final problem with psychiatric diagnoses is that they can affect how we perceive, or misperceive, the people who have been given them. Studies (Martinez et al., 2011; Read & Harper, 2022; Read et al., 2013a; Wright et al., 2011) have found that, when we apply a psychiatric diagnostic label to someone, we are more likely to:

- expect them to be dangerous
- think they are unpredictable
- not believe they are responsible for their actions
- perceive them to have less 'humanity'
- think their problem is severe
- think they are unlikely to recover from their problems
- be frightened of them
- reject them and want to keep a distance.

We will revisit stigma and prejudice in the next chapter.

Conclusions

We make no apologies for repeating ourselves (again!) in this conclusion. The power of the labels we use in everyday life is huge, especially when we invest with any authority the person or institution doing the labelling. And when we, the labelled, are in a position of weakness and vulnerability (perhaps frightened and desperate for help), the process becomes very hard to challenge. A further problem is that, since the whole of life is becoming medicalised, we fail to notice the flimsy reliability and validity of the labels. It has become a given, taken for granted – a fact about the world that we can only think from, rather than think about. French sociologist Pierre Bourdieu captures it when he says: 'It goes without saying because it comes without saying'(1977, p.167). Furthermore, any critical voices are often denigrated (labelled, or 'diagnosed') as 'antipsychiatry', irresponsible, troublemaking, dangerous, unscientific or extremist (Davies, 2022; Taylor-Page, 2022).

The main point of all of this, in a book about the causes of mental health problems, is that, contrary to what we might hope, a psychiatric diagnosis does not help us understand what is going on at all. And if we swallow the idea that we 'have' some sort of 'disorder' or 'illness' inside us, the diagnosis can actually mask the real causes of our problems – which we, and many others, argue lie in the events and circumstances of our lives. Furthermore, such acceptance of the power of diagnosis disempowers us, since it can stop us believing that we can do anything to make things better ourselves. After all, if you are one of those people who happen to 'have' a 'depressive disorder' (in your brain or your genes, or both), then there isn't too much you can really do about it (other than take your medication for life). But if you realise that your sometimes feeling depressed is largely a reaction to depressing things happening, then maybe, with help if necessary, you can do something to avoid more depressing things happening or to change how you are reacting to them.

If you like having a label to sum up all the complexities of what is happening to you or your loved one, then by all means hang on to your diagnosis. If, on the other hand, you want to try figuring out where the problem actually started and what is maintaining it, and are even willing to try something new in an effort to make things better, then it's probably best not to pay too much attention to your diagnosis. And, of course, you can always do both if that's what works best for you, since it's not just a slogan when we say everyone is different and requires a unique approach. It's a fact.

Chapter 5
Public opinion: depression is caused by depressing things happening

While we 'experts' continue to argue about the causes of mental health problems, the public have already voted. In research surveys all over the world, the result is the same: the vast majority of people think that social causes explain mental distress (however severe or enduring) better than biological causes.

In 22 of 23 countries where research surveys have been conducted, the public believe that things like poverty, family stress, loneliness, relationship problems, child abuse, loss, war trauma and so forth are more important causes of 'schizophrenia' or psychosis than biological factors like genetics or chemical imbalances. 'Schizophrenia' is often supposed to be the most biogenetically based 'mental illness', and yet the public believe its origins are psychosocial. A few mental health professionals still claim that the idea that bad things happen and screw us up is very controversial. But it seems it is only controversial to a numerically tiny sector of the mental health world – primarily biologically oriented psychiatrists and drug company executives.

The list of countries is Australia, Bali, Brazil, Canada, China, England, Ethiopia, France, Germany, Greece, India, Ireland, Italy, Japan, Malaysia, Mongolia, New Zealand, Nigeria, Russia, South Africa, Switzerland and Turkey (Read et al., 2006, 2013b). The exception is the USA, which has an extremely biomedical mental health system that is heavily influenced by drug companies. Here, public opinion is more equally divided between biogenetic and psychosocial. We should note that, in six countries, spiritual explanations were more popular than either social or biological ones (Read et al., 2013b).

Most of these surveys allow respondents to choose more than one explanation rather than just choose between social and biological. Often there is quite a long list of possible causes to choose from. This reveals that the public actually take a quite sophisticated approach to the causes of mental health problems. They certainly recognise both social and biological causes, adopting what the experts would call a 'multifactorial' approach. There is, however, a very strong pattern in terms of what sorts of causes they think are most important. In all 22 countries, social causes easily beat biological illness-type causes (Read et al., 2013b).

We'll look at just a few of the many studies demonstrating that, for many years now, the public has understood that human distress is primarily caused by our social environment. Some surveys ask about the causes of mental health problems in general and others focus on the causes of specific problems, usually either depression or 'schizophrenia'.

In England, a survey found that, in relation to mental health in general:

> Life events, family problems and economic hardship were mentioned frequently, with genetic and biological causes noted much less frequently. (Rogers & Pilgrim, 1997)

When Londoners were asked specifically about schizophrenia:

> Overall subjects seemed to prefer environmental explanations referring to social stressors and family conflicts – e.g. 'being mercilessly persecuted by family and friends' and 'having come from backgrounds that promote stress'. (Furnham & Rees, 1988)

Another London study found that the most endorsed causal model of schizophrenia was 'unusual or traumatic experiences or the failure to negotiate some critical stage of emotional development', followed by 'social, economic, and family pressures'. The researchers concluded:

> It seems that lay people have not been converted to the medical view and prefer psychosocial explanations... Subjects agreed that schizophrenic behaviour had some meaning and was neither random nor simply a symptom of an illness. (Furnham & Bower, 1992)

An Irish survey found that the most commonly cited causes for the positive symptoms of schizophrenia (e.g. hallucinations and delusions) were stressful life events. Only 11% cited biogenetic causes. For negative symptoms (e.g. social withdrawal), the most frequently cited cause was childhood problems such as 'lack of adequate parental love' (Barry & Greene, 1992). Only 5% cited biogenetic causes.

A 2013 survey of 900 Australians found that the two most endorsed causes of depression were 'day-to-day-problems such as stress, family arguments, difficulties at work or financial difficulties' and 'the recent death of a close friend or relative' (both 97%), followed by 'recent traumatic events' and 'problems from childhood such as being badly treated or abused, losing one or both parents when young or coming from a broken home' (96%) (Pilkington et al., 2013).

The most comprehensive series of large-scale national surveys has been conducted over many years in Germany. When the researchers reviewed all their studies, they concluded that, for both depression and schizophrenia, 'acute stress in the form of life events is the most frequently endorsed cause, followed by chronic stress in partnership and family' (Angermeyer & Dietrich, 2006).

'Patients'

Since people who use mental health services are members of the public, it should come as no surprise that they also understand their problems in terms of what has gone on in their lives, more than in terms of genes and neurotransmitters. Since the turn of the century, numerous books (Geekie & Read, 2009; Geekie et al., 2011; Romme et al., 2009) and journal articles (Bullimore, 2010; Dillon, 2010) have ended decades of ignoring what people diagnosed with psychotic disorders like 'schizophrenia' have to say about their own experiences and what might have caused them. While a vast array of causes is cited, showing again that everyone is different, many write about bad childhood experiences that they believe contributed to their difficulties in adulthood.

A USA study of four 'stakeholder groups' concluded, in relation to 'schizophrenia', that patients, family members and the public endorsed 'factors consistent with a non-biomedical view of mental illness more frequently than did the clinicians' (van Dorn et al., 2005). Patients were most likely (66%) and clinicians least likely (18%) to cite 'the way he was raised' as a cause. Clinicians were significantly more likely to endorse genetics as a cause than the other three groups, and patients were less likely than clinicians to endorse chemical imbalance. 'Stressful circumstances' was cited significantly more often by both patients and family members than by clinicians.

A 2013 review of available research found that all 16 samples of people diagnosed with 'schizophrenia' from nine countries (including the USA) cited life events as being more important than biogenetic causes (Read et al., 2013b). For example, the causes espoused as 'likely/very likely' by Germans who experienced psychosis were: 'recent psychosocial factors' – 88%; 'personality' – 71%; 'family' – 64%, and 'biology' – 31% (Holzinger et al, 2002). Indeed, the German 'patients' endorsed 'psychosocial stress factors' even more strongly than the rest of the population. In an Italian study of people diagnosed with 'schizophrenia', 76% mentioned at least one social cause, with 10% citing a biological cause (Magliano et al., 2009).

A study in London (Pistrang & Barker, 1992) found that only 5% of people diagnosed as 'schizophrenic' believed that their problems were a result of having a 'mental illness', and 13% cited other biological causes, but 43% cited social causes such as interpersonal problems, stress and childhood events. Another London study found that African-Caribbean, Bangladeshi and West African people diagnosed with 'schizophrenia' had even more psychosocial and spiritual causal beliefs than their white counterparts and were less likely to endorse biological causes (McCabe & Priebe, 2004).

The largest ever survey of causal beliefs among people taking antidepressants (1,829 participants) found that the most frequently endorsed beliefs about what causes depression were family stress, relationship problems, loss of a loved one, financial problems, isolation, and abuse or neglect in childhood (Read et al., 2014b).

In a more recent survey, 701 people from 30 countries who were prescribed antipsychotic medication were asked an open question about what had caused the problems for which they were taking the drugs (Read, 2020). On a scale from 1 = 'purely biological' to 5 = 'purely social', the mean score for their responses was 4.2. Analysis of their 1,063 causal statements produced seven themes: social (49.9%), psychological (12.1%), biogenetic (11.6%), iatrogenic (caused by the treatments) (11.3%), drug and alcohol (6.7%), medical condition (4.5%) and insomnia (4.0%). Respondents were 13 times more likely to report predominantly or exclusively social causes than they did predominantly or exclusively biogenetic causes.

A sensible response to these findings might be, 'Well, they should know'. But 'Not at all!' say some psychiatrists. These people's belief that they have been driven mad by awful things happening to them is still sometimes dismissed by professionals as a lack of 'insight' into the fact that they have an 'illness'. Some psychiatrists even use this supposed lack of insight as a diagnostic indicator that their 'patients' are still ill. To be seen as recovered, it seems a person has to admit that they were wrong to think that their problems are related to their life circumstances. They have to agree with the psychiatrist's opinion that they have a biologically based illness. Some psychiatrists have gone so far as to argue that choosing not to believe in biological psychiatry's illness model is not only a symptom of 'schizophrenia', it is a specific 'neurological deficit', which they have called 'anosognosia' (Read, 2020).

This notion that a specific malfunction in the brain causes you to not believe in an illness explanation for your difficulties is a powerful example of how dominant, and silly, the 'medical model' has become. The original (psychoanalytic) meaning of 'insight' was in fact the ability to understand your current difficulties in relation to past life events, especially those in childhood. Now, for some psychiatrists, it means exactly the opposite.

Family members

If you were to rely entirely on the internet and the media to find out what the relatives of people who use mental health services think, you might conclude that most family members strongly endorse the illness model and want to see their 'sick' relatives permanently on medication or kept in hospital. It turns out that the so-called 'family organisations' that are often quoted or invited to speak on news and current affairs programmes are heavily sponsored by drug companies. Organisations such as SANE in the UK, NAMI (National Alliance for the Mentally Ill) in the USA, and the Schizophrenia Society of Canada, which receive so much media coverage, are not at all representative of family members in general (Read & Magliano, 2011; Read et al., 2013b).

We have already mentioned the 2005 USA study that showed that both 'patients' and their relatives have, like the general public, a far more psychosocial framework than mental health professionals. Numerous other studies have shown that relatives of mental health service users elsewhere in the world also share the beliefs of the general public. This is true even for that supposedly biological illness 'schizophrenia'. As early as 1988, the German researchers mentioned earlier cited five international studies showing that the relatives of 'schizophrenics' believed that the causes were social, and they went on to find the same among German relatives (Angermeyer et al., 1988).

The 2013 review mentioned earlier (Read et al., 2013b) found that 19 of 24 surveys of the families of people diagnosed 'schizophrenic' endorsed social causes more than biological ones. If the USA studies are excluded, the proportion becomes 14 out of 15. For example, an Italian survey of 709 relatives of people diagnosed 'schizophrenic' found that the most commonly endorsed causes were 'stress' and 'psychological traumas', with 68% of them believing that schizophrenia is caused entirely by psychosocial factors (Magliano et al., 2004). The finding is consistent across a range of cultures. Relatives in Turkey cited stressful events (50%) and family conflicts (40%) more often than biological/genetic factors (23%) (Karanci, 1995). Similarly, 55% of Indian relatives cited social stressors, whereas only 5% cited heredity and 14% brain disorder (Srinivasan & Thara, 2001).

Studies conducted since the review by Read and colleagues (2013b) tend to produce similar findings. For example, a 2019 study of 350 'primary caregivers' in Singapore found:

> The majority of caregivers identified psychosocial causes, followed by biological, supernatural, and lastly drug-/substance use-related causes for their relatives' illness'.
> (Sagayadevan et al., 2020)

Further evidence of relatives' rejection of biogenetic beliefs comes from research into 'psychoeducation' programmes specifically designed to teach them the illness model. One study assessed relatives' retention of 'knowledge' about the 'illness' and found 'absolutely no change in the amount of knowledge between pretests and posttests' (Cozolino et al., 1988). Another found that, before psychoeducation, just 11% of relatives believed the problems were caused by a 'disordered brain', and, having had the training, still only 32% believed it, while belief in 'genetic inheritance' increased from 11% to 15%. Just 3% of the patients adopted an illness model, before or after the programme (McGill et al., 1983).

Prejudice: another major contributor to mental health problems

The ill-informed and frequently unpleasant stereotypes that some people hold (and are all exposed to) about people with mental health problems cannot, of course, cause the problems in the first place. Nevertheless, prejudice is a huge factor in preventing people from recovering from their difficulties. This is especially true if you internalise the negative attitudes and really start believing that you are inferior, useless, damaged or even dangerous. In Chapter 7, we will see that the cognitive model argues that what we tell ourselves about ourselves is a major cause and maintainer of things like depression. If we are faced with negative attitudes from some members of the public (and some mental health staff), it can be even harder to start replacing our existing negative thoughts with more positive ones. This is a serious issue. Prejudice against people with mental health problems is not just a set of privately held attitudes. Research has found that the prejudice is often acted on in terms of blatant discrimination in, for instance, employment and housing. The stereotypes for people deemed to be 'schizophrenic' are the worst of all, with dangerousness and unpredictability at the core of a very toxic set of beliefs (Read et al., 2013a).

Although not directly relevant to our thinking about the causes of mental health problems, it is interesting to note how psychiatry has responded to all this prejudice and discrimination. Most 'destigmatisation' programmes around the world, which are often funded by drug companies, have adopted the approach of trying to 'educate' us that we are wrong to believe that our problems are caused by events in our lives, and to persuade us instead that we have an 'illness' caused by some kind of biochemical imbalance. This 'mental illness is an illness like any other' approach to reducing prejudice is based on the idea that, if a person is ill, they cannot be held responsible for their actions and therefore cannot be blamed. This is well-intentioned, but wrong.

Almost all the research investigating the relationship between what we believe about causes and how prejudiced we are goes in the opposite direction (Longden & Read, 2017; Read & Harper, 2022). One review found that in 28 of 31 studies (90%), biogenetic causal beliefs were related to negative attitudes, and that in 24 of 26 studies (92%), psychosocial beliefs were related to positive attitudes (Read et al., 2013a). Two other reviews have found, more specifically, that biogenetic beliefs are related to the belief that people with mental health problems are dangerous, to a desire for distance from them, and to pessimism about their recovery (Kvaale et al., 2013a, 2013b)

Here is just one example. A research student of John's made a video (like those used in professional training courses) of a young man (an actor) talking about hearing voices and believing that everyone was out to get him. He showed the video to three groups of young people, and then a doctor gave an explanation of the causes of these 'symptoms'. However the doctor gave a different explanation to each of the groups. The first group was told these were symptoms of the brain disease 'schizophrenia'; the second was told the symptoms were caused by a combination of biological and social factors, and the third was told that the voices and paranoia were reactions to trauma in the person's life. Attitudes were measured before and after the videos. In the first group (brain disease, schizophrenia) perceptions of 'dangerousness' and 'unpredictability' significantly increased. For the other two groups, these negative attitudes decreased (Walker & Read, 2002).

This relationship between bio-genetic causal beliefs and negative attitudes exists among mental health professionals too (Larkings & Brown, 2018). In one study, 343 US mental health staff read descriptions of patients diagnosed with four 'disorders' and were given biogenetic or psychosocial explanations. For example, the psychosocial explanation for social phobia was bullying, neglectful parents and failure to learn to trust others, while the biogenetic account was low serotonin levels, abnormally active amygdala and a hereditary component. The staff who were given the biological explanations showed significantly lower levels of empathy towards the patients, across all four conditions (Lebowitz & Ahn, 2014).

The relationship also holds for people who have been given the diagnosis: those who espouse a more biological explanation for their difficulties engage in more 'self-stigma' or 'internalized stigma' (Carter et al., 2017; Larkings & Brown, 2018; Read et al., 2013a).

It doesn't help, it seems, to persuade us that the brains and genes of people who are struggling to cope are somehow different from those of the rest of us. Research from other fields about how to combat prejudice tells us that you have to emphasise similarities, not differences. And when your strategy to reduce the prejudice and stigma includes telling people that the differences are due to unchangeable brain abnormalities or defective genes, then it is hardly surprising that this approach actually makes it worse. (Readers wanting to find out more about exactly why and how this approach impacts our attitudes should do an internet search for the keyword 'essentialism' (Haslam et al., 2006; Kvalle et al., 2013a, 2013b).)

Biological psychiatrists have been trying for more than half a century to get us to think like them. In 1961 the US Joint Commission on Mental Illness and Health concluded:

> The principle of sameness as applied to the mentally sick versus the physically sick has become a cardinal tenet of mental health education… Psychiatry has tried diligently to make society see the mentally ill in its way and has railed at the public's antipathy or indifference. (Joint Commission on Mental Illness and Health, 1961)

We have known for more than two decades that this approach increases rather than decreases prejudice. It makes sense, of course, that the drug companies would disregard this and continue to spend millions on 'destigmatisation' campaigns that continue to push the illness model. But it seems unfortunate that some mental health professionals go along with it. It is certainly unscientific.

What the public believes is, of course, just a set of beliefs, not 'scientific fact'. But the same is true of the tiny numbers of people – mostly biological psychiatrists and drug company executives – who believe the opposite. We shall see in the next chapter whether the research tends to support the ideas of the majority or the ideas of the minority.

What does seem to be a fact is that, despite a concerted attempt, spanning 70 years or so and involving huge amounts of money, to persuade us that we are wrong to focus on the obvious, social causes of our problems – the ones we might be able to do something about – we remain unconvinced.

Chapter 6
Is the public right? What does the research say about the causes of mental health problems?

In the previous chapter, we looked at the research surveying the views of non-professionals, including patients and family members. Survey respondents in different countries consistently identify the social causes of mental health problems, including:

In the UK
- life events, family problems and economic hardship
- social stressors and family conflicts – e.g., being mercilessly persecuted by family and friends
- having come from backgrounds that promote stress
- unusual or traumatic experiences
- social, economic, and family pressures.

In Australia
- day-to-day-problems such as stress, family arguments, difficulties at work or financial difficulties
- the recent death of a close friend or relative
- traumatic events
- problems from childhood such as being badly treated or abused, losing one or both parents when young or coming from a broken home.

In Ireland
- stressful life events
- childhood problems such as lack of adequate parental love

In Germany
- acute stress in the form of life events
- chronic stress in partnership and family

In the USA
- the way the person was raised
- stressful circumstances.

The public seem to recognise two general groups of social causes: past and present (or recent). The causes in the past tend to focus, unsurprisingly, on childhood. The causes in the present are ongoing stresses of various sorts. Some specific types of causes, some of which span past and present, childhood and adulthood, are poverty, trauma/abuse/violence, neglect, loss and general day-to-day stress.

Does research support these widely held public beliefs? The research summarised next focuses largely, but not only, on the more extreme mental health problems like psychosis and 'schizophrenia'. This is mainly because, if we can demonstrate that something as supposedly biological as 'schizophrenia' is actually largely caused by social factors, then it should not be surprising that things like depression and anxiety are also primarily caused by things that happen in our lives. We will pay more attention to depression in Chapter 8.

It should be stressed from the outset that it is usually a combination of the factors discussed here, rather than any one of them in isolation, that tend to tip people into the kinds of distressing experiences that are likely to be diagnosed as psychosis or any other mental health problem (Cromby et al., 2013d). Poverty by itself, for example, rarely causes mental health problems. However, in combination with childhood neglect, for example, which is more likely if you grow up in a poor family, your chances of becoming extremely depressed are relatively high compared with someone who grows up in a safe, nurturing, relatively well-off family. Furthermore, the richer you are, the more resources, professional or otherwise, you have at your disposal to help you through emotionally difficult times. Stressed, rich people take their holidays on super-yachts, while the rest of us take our breaks in the loony bin. Or so an old joke says.

Poverty

Mental hospitals have been filled predominantly with poor people throughout history. In Chapter 2 we saw, for example, that the people confined in the Hôpital Général in 17th-century Paris were 'the poor of Paris'. A study conducted in Chicago in 1939 found that there were higher psychiatric admission rates in the deprived central areas of the city than in the wealthier suburbs. Contrary to the notion that milder mental health problems are socially caused, but not 'schizophrenia', the study found that people in the poorest areas of Chicago were seven times more likely to be diagnosed 'schizophrenic' than those in the richest parts (Read et al., 2013c). This relationship between poverty and a diagnosis of 'schizophrenia' was quickly replicated in nine other cities throughout the USA. During the 1950s, the same relationship was found in Bristol, Liverpool, London and in Norway (Kohn, 1976).

A famous US study (Hollingshead & Redlich, 1954) found that people in the poorest class (V – 'unskilled, manual') were three times more likely than those in the wealthiest two classes (I & II – 'business, professional and managerial') to be treated for psychiatric problems in general. The diagnosis with the strongest relationship with class was, again, 'schizophrenia'. The poorest people were eight times more likely to be diagnosed as 'schizophrenic' than the wealthiest.

By 1976 a review concluded:

> There have been more than 50 studies of the relationship between social class and rates of 'schizophrenia'. Almost without exception, these studies have shown that 'schizophrenia' occurs most frequently at the lowest social class levels of urban society. The evidence comes from research in Canada, Denmark, Finland, Great Britain, Norway, Sweden, Taiwan, and the United States – an unusually large number of countries and cultures for establishing the generality of any relationship in social science. (Kohn, 1976)

A 1980 New York study of first admissions found that people in social class V were 12 times more likely to be hospitalised than those in social class I, while a Tennessee study of 10,000 first admissions confirmed that 'schizophrenia' was the diagnosis most strongly related to socio-economic status. The relationship between 'schizophrenia' and poverty was described as 'one of the most consistent findings in the field of psychiatric epidemiology' (Eaton, 1980).

Since 1980, the relationship between poverty and being admitted to a psychiatric hospital has been confirmed repeatedly, in Bristol, London, Nottingham, Wales, Finland, New Zealand, Canada, Nigeria, Israel, the USA, (Read, 2010; Read et al., 2013c), Scotland (McCartney et al., 2013) and Finland (Suokas et al., 2019). More often than not, the strongest relationship between class and psychiatric admission is for the diagnosis of 'schizophrenia' (Read, 2010; Read et al., 2013c).

For example, a British study found that deprived children are four times more likely to develop 'non-schizophrenic psychotic illness' but eight times more likely to grow up to be 'schizophrenic' than non-deprived children (Harrison et al., 2001). Even among children with no family history of psychosis, deprived children were seven times more likely to develop 'schizophrenia', which questions the whole idea of a genetic predisposition.

While poverty is particularly predictive of a 'schizophrenia' diagnosis (Read, 2010), it is also predictive of a host of other mental health problems, including depression, generalised anxiety disorders, phobias, panic disorder, alcohol abuse, drug abuse, erectile dysfunction, and childhood 'disorders' such as 'conduct disorder'. For example, a study covering 14 USA states found that admission to hospital for depression was significantly predicted by both poverty and unemployment (Fortney et al., 2007). A British study that had followed nearly 10,000 adults since their birth found that those who were poor at age 7 were significantly more likely at age 45 to have generalised anxiety disorder, depressive episodes, phobias and panic disorder (Stansfield et al., 2008). A more recent investigation by Public Health England found that antidepressants were prescribed in the most deprived 20% of neighbourhoods at 'a markedly increased rate' compared with the wealthiest 20% (Taylor et al., 2019).

As mentioned above, poverty itself may not be a direct cause of mental health problems, but it increases the chances of exposure to things that are direct causes, which is why poverty is sometimes called 'the cause of the causes'. A good example of this is a recent study of 3,500 65–75-year-old New Yorkers, which found that living in a poor neighbourhood predicted depression levels, but that this relationship was largely explained by the high levels of violence in the locality (Joshi et al., 2017).

Relative poverty

There is also convincing evidence that *relative* poverty is a stronger predictor than absolute poverty *per se*. Relative poverty is usually measured by the difference in income between the wealthiest 10% and the poorest 10% of a population. In their book *The Spirit Level*,[1] British epidemiologists Richard Wilkinson and Kate Pickett report multiple studies demonstrating an even stronger relationship between relative poverty and a range of social, health and mental health outcomes than between poverty *per se* and the same outcomes (Wilkinson & Pickett, 2009). They first note that in many countries rates of 'mental illness' and levels of inequality have both increased significantly in recent decades. They then report a strong relationship between degree of income inequality and rates of people meeting diagnostic criteria for mental illness over a 12-month period, across 12 countries (see Figure 6.1).

Similar findings are reported for other outcomes, including level of use of illegal drugs (Figure 6.2).

Urbanicity

Growing up or living in large cites is also a factor in a wide range of mental health problems, including depression and substance abuse. Again, the relationship is even stronger for 'schizophrenia' than for other diagnoses (Read, 2010; Read et al., 2013c). Not only is being diagnosed 'schizophrenic' associated with living in urban areas, but the greater the numbers of years lived in urban areas prior to diagnosis, the greater the risk of being diagnosed 'schizophrenic' later in life (Pedersen & Mortensen, 2001).

---

1. See also www.equalitytrust.org.uk

74   *A Straight Talking Introduction to the Causes of Mental Health Problems*

**Figure 6.1:
The prevalence of mental illness is higher in more unequal rich countries**
Source: Wilkinson & Pickett (2009). *The Spirit Level.* Allen Lane.

Reproduced by kind permission of The Equality Trust
www.equalitytrust.org.uk

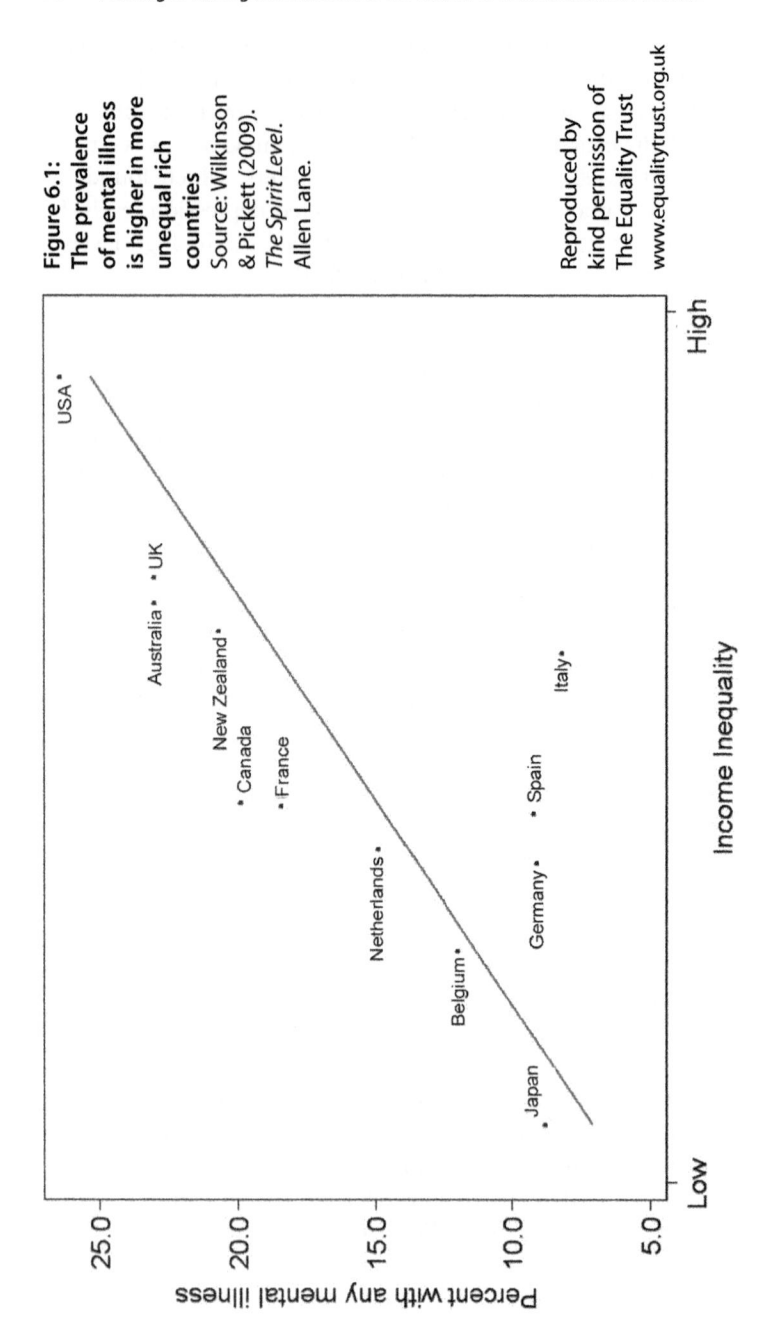

What does the research say about the causes of mental health problems? 75

**Figure 6.2:
Drug use is more common in unequal countries (opiates, cocaine, cannabis, ecstasy, amphetamines)**
Source: Wilkinson & Pickett (2009). *The Spirit Level.* Allen Lane.

Reproduced by kind permission of The Equality Trust
www.equalitytrust.org.uk

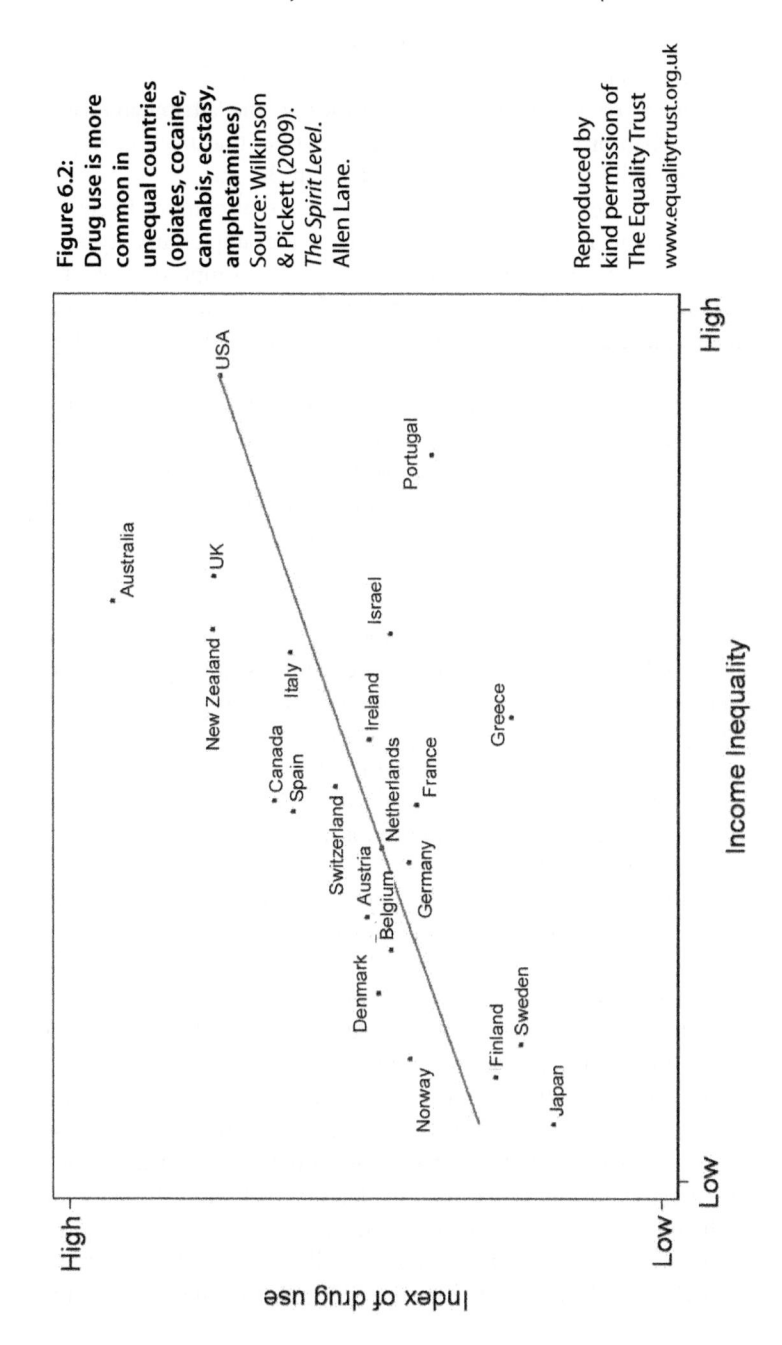

The relationship between urban living and 'schizophrenia' remains after controlling for family history of psychiatric disorder in general, or of 'schizophrenia' specifically. The 'attributable risk' from urban birth was four times greater than that from having a mother with 'schizophrenia' (Read et al., 2013c).

Most other mental health problems are also more likely to occur if you live in a city, including, for example, anxiety and PTSD (Ventimiglia & Seedat, 2019). The complexity of the interactions between various social and cultural factors is, again, nicely illustrated by a recent review of research on the relationship between urban living and depression (Sampson et al., 2020). While several studies found the expected relationship, in two studies it came down to how much green space there was in various neighbourhoods, rather than poverty *per se*. Furthermore, three studies in China found that living in the city had some protective factors against depression that living in rural China did not.

Ethnicity

The relationship between ethnicity and mental health problems is complex and hotly debated. The demonstrated relationship between a range of mental health problems and belonging to indigenous groups, colonised people or ethnic minorities seems to have little or nothing to do with the race, ethnicity or culture itself and everything to do with the social circumstances in which many members of such groups are forced to live, including discrimination and poverty.

Ethnicity is a powerful predictor of a diagnosis of 'schizophrenia'. This has been demonstrated in Australia, Belgium, Denmark, Germany, Greenland, the Netherlands, New Zealand, Israel, Sweden, the UK and the USA (Read et al., 2013c). In the UK, for example, the incidence rates for 'schizophrenia' are 3.6 times higher among all ethnic minority groups combined than among whites. In the UK, Afro-Caribbeans have been found to be nine to 12 times more likely to be diagnosed 'schizophrenic' than white people (Read et al., 2013c). Although racist misdiagnoses are part of the explanation, the factors that link ethnicity to 'schizophrenia' are poverty, unemployment, discrimination and social isolation. Janssen and colleagues (2003) recorded experiences of discrimination in 4,067 Dutch people. Those who had reported discrimination in two or more domains (skin colour/ethnicity, gender, age and so on) were three times more likely to be experiencing psychotic hallucinations than those who had reported no discrimination, and five times more likely to be experiencing psychotic delusions. A study of more than 10,000 Swedes looked at a range of problems, including depression, and concluded that 'the association between immigrant status and mental illness appears above all to be an effect of a higher prevalence of social and economic disadvantage' (Tinhog et al., 2007).

Gender

Most mental health problems are diagnosed in women far more often than in men, including the two most common – depression and anxiety – as well as eating disorders, borderline personality disorders, post-traumatic disorder and so on. Women are about twice as likely be prescribed antidepressants (Taylor et al., 2019) and electroconvulsive therapy (ECT) (Read et al., 2019, 2021) than men. Space does not permit a full discussion of why all this is the case (Taylor, 2022; Tseris, 2020; Read & Beavan, 2013) but suffice it to say that the differences are largely explained by women disproportionately suffering some of the main causes of these problems, such as poverty, childhood sexual abuse, rape, partner violence and so on. The continuing influence of gender roles is illustrated, however, by the fact that two diagnoses given more often to men are substance abuse disorders and antisocial personality disorder (Cromby et al., 2013d).

Trauma

The public, as we have seen, have no difficulty grasping that mental health problems tend to be caused primarily by bad things happening to us. Even the American Psychiatric Association has included 'post-traumatic stress disorder' (PTSD) in the *DSM* (see Chapter 4) – which it did in 1968. Interestingly, this diagnosis (the only one in the *DSM* to acknowledge the social cause of a problem in its name) was not formally recognised in response to the effects of violence against children and women; it entered the *DSM* because of the thousands of Vietnam war veterans returning to the USA in a traumatised state, many of whom killed themselves (Schlenger et al., 2015).

Traumatic events, however, contribute to a much wider range of mental health problems than PTSD, including the most common ones, like depression and anxiety disorders. There is now a significant, wide-ranging and undeniable body of research documenting that the public are right when they think that things like child abuse, rape and violent assaults in adulthood, war traumas and so on are extremely powerful factors in a vast array of mental health problems. There is space to summarise only a tiny fraction of this research here.

Of course, not everyone exposed to abuse or violence ends up having terrifying, disabling experiences and a mental health diagnosis. Research and common sense tell us that the best indicators of which abused/assaulted people end up in a bad state are:

- if the abuse occurs early in life
- if there are multiple incidents or types of abuse
- if it is inflicted by a loved one on whom we are dependent
- in the case of child abuse, whether we managed to tell someone soon afterwards and were believed and supported, rather than told to keep it a secret or that it did not happen.

Child abuse

A review of 59 studies of the most severely disturbed people receiving psychiatric treatment found that 64% of the women and 55% of the men had been physically or sexually abused as children (Read et al., 2008). Most of the physical abuse was inflicted by family members. For more than half of the sexually abused females and about a quarter of the sexually abused males, the abuser was a family member (incest) (Read et al., 2005).

Psychiatric patients subjected to childhood sexual or physical abuse have earlier first admissions to hospital, longer and more frequent hospitalisations, spend longer in seclusion, receive more medication, are more likely to self-mutilate, and have higher global symptom severity (Larkin & Morrison, 2006; Read et al., 2008).

Psychiatric patients who were abused as children are also far more likely to try to kill themselves. Two New Zealand studies, one a general population study and one a clinical sample, illustrate the strength of the relationship between child abuse and suicidality. A survey of more than 2,000 women found that those who had been sexually abused as children were 19 times more likely to have tried to kill themselves (and seven times more likely to have been admitted to a psychiatric hospital). Those who had been physically abused were five times more likely to have tried to take their own life (Mullen et al., 1993). A study of 200 adult psychiatric outpatients found that child abuse (on average about 20 years earlier) was a better predictor of current suicidality than a current diagnosis of depression (Read et al., 2001b).

Child abuse is now known to have a significant causal role in most mental health problems, including depression, anxiety disorders, PTSD, eating disorders, sexual difficulties, substance abuse, personality disorders, and dissociative disorders.

Child neglect and emotional abuse

More subtle, ongoing childhood circumstances can be just as damaging to our long-term mental health as more blatant events like being sexually attacked or repeatedly beaten. The absence of love ('emotional neglect') or of the basics of life ('physical neglect'), or being repeatedly told you are 'rubbish' or 'useless' ('emotional abuse') have all, unsurprisingly, been linked to a whole range of mental health problems later in life.

The survey of 2,000 New Zealand women (Mullen et al., 1993) found that those who had been emotionally abused were three times more likely to be depressed or to have sexual problems, four times more likely to have an eating disorder, five times more likely to have had a psychiatric admission and 12 times more likely to have tried to end their own life. Studies elsewhere around the world produce similar results. The 2008 review by Read and colleagues mentioned above found, in six studies of adults diagnosed 'schizophrenic', the following average rates: emotional neglect – 51%; physical neglect – 41%, and emotional abuse – 47%.

Bullying

Being repeatedly picked on or beaten up at school (and the added humiliation these days of having the incidents broadcast on social media) can, obviously, lower our self-esteem, lead to depression, destroy our trust in other people in general, and, at its extreme, lead (understandably) to paranoia. People in England who were bullied as children or adolescents have been found to be up to four times more likely to be diagnosed as psychotic later in life (Bebbington et al., 2004).

Adverse childhood experiences

Nowadays, studies tend to include a broad range of childhood adversities, or 'adverse childhood experiences' (ACEs) (Felitti et al., 1998), rather than specific types of abuse or neglect. For example, a survey of 850 first-year students at one university found the number of childhood adversities (measured by the 10-item ACEs scale) was significantly associated with higher levels of anxiety and lower levels of physical and mental health and overall 'quality of life' (Davies et al., 2021).

In 2012, the first meta-analysis of studies investigating the relationship between childhood adversities and psychosis was published (Varese et al., 2012). A meta-analysis goes beyond ordinary research reviews in that it includes only the most rigorous studies and combines their results, allowing for differences in sample sizes and methodologies. The 2012 meta-analysis included only the 41 best designed studies of the 736 screened. Analysing these 41 studies together revealed that people who had suffered one or more childhood adversities were 2.8 times more likely to develop psychosis than were those who had not. The meta-analysis also generated odds ratios for six types of adversity separately: sexual abuse, 2.4; physical abuse, 2.9; emotional abuse, 3.4; neglect, 2.9; bullying, 2.4; parental death, 1.7.

Nine of the ten studies that tested for a 'dose-response' found that the greater the exposure to adverse events, the more likely the person was to be diagnosed with a psychotic disorder. For example, a UK survey of 8,580 people found that those subjected to one form of adverse event were 1.7 times more likely to be diagnosed with a psychotic disorder, rising to 18 times more likely for three adverse events and 193 times for five types (Shevlin et al., 2007).[2]

---

2. To watch a 2005 public debate at the Institute of Psychiatry in London where John proposed the motion that 'Child abuse is a cause of schizophrenia', go to: www.kcl.ac.uk/maudsley-debates-21st-to-30th

Rape and violence in adulthood

Being raped or physically assaulted is most obviously connected to PTSD. The three major 'symptom' groups of PTSD are heightened vigilance, re-experiencing symptoms (flashbacks, dreams and so on) and avoidance (of certain social situations and of feelings – 'numbing'). These 'symptoms' become perfectly understandable once the trauma (rape, assault and so on) is known about. Again, however, our diagnostic system – designed to put people into boxes – often masks the fact that interpersonal violence can also lead to a whole range of other difficulties, including depression, phobias, dissociative disorders and, yet again, psychosis.

Most psychiatric patients suffer serious assaults as adults. It is sometimes difficult to determine which comes first: the violence or the unusual behaviour or stigma that might have prompted the violence. It is also true that, when severely disturbed, we can be particularly vulnerable to predators and others inclined to violence (Larkin & Morrison, 2006). One study found that 63% of people receiving psychiatric outpatient treatment had suffered violence by family members in the previous year, compared with 35% in the general population. Some 69% of the women and 49% of the men reported adulthood domestic violence; 40% of the women had suffered rape or attempted rape in adulthood, of whom 53% had attempted suicide as a result (in the general population, the comparable rates are 7% of women, of whom 3% have attempted suicide), and 12% of men with severe mental illness had been seriously sexually assaulted, compared with 0.5% in the general population (Khalifeh et al., 2015).

War trauma

Seeing people killed, while your own life is simultaneously at risk, can lead to PTSD and also to a range of other severe difficulties (Schlenger et al., 2015). Again, this includes psychosis, and research studies have found this link not just in combat veterans but also in prisoners of war, war-rape victims, refugees from the Pol Pot regime and from war in Somalia, people exposed to bombings, shootings and 'punishment' beatings in Northern Ireland, and Holocaust survivors (Larkin & Morrison, 2006; Larkin & Read, 2008; Read et al., 2008). More recently, high rates of PTSD and 'other severe mental disorders' have been found in combatants and civilians in the wars in Syria (Kakaje et al., 2021) and Ukraine (Johnson et al., 2022).

Loss

Losing a loved one can, of course, fall into the category of 'trauma'. We have given it its own section, however, because loss, in its various forms, is such a huge cause of mental health problems and because, like child abuse, it sometimes doesn't receive the attention it deserves, especially from those mental health professionals who see our problems as biologically based 'illnesses'.

Like poverty, loss by itself does not necessarily lead to mental health problems. The sadness we feel when mourning the death of a loved one is not a mental health problem (although some doctors are happy to 'treat' it as such by prescribing antidepressants or tranquillisers). As discussed earlier, a combination of factors is usually required before we get into serious emotional difficulties. Three of the more obvious factors that can influence whether we come through a period of mourning in relatively good shape after a loss are:

1. whether we have recently experienced other significant losses
2. how much support and understanding we get while mourning
3. how close we were to the loved one who has died.

A fourth exacerbating factor is being told by a professional that your sadness is a sign of some kind of mental illness, such as a 'depressive disorder'. This can both invalidate your feelings and make you worry that there is something seriously and irreversibly wrong with you for feeling so down. This can interfere with the natural grieving process and, ironically, help lock you into a longer period of depression than if you had just been left with your normal social supports. 'Time is a great healer' is a cliché, but it's often true.

Given the increasing medicalisation of everything in life, mental health professionals who confuse grieving with 'mental illness' are not helped by research, often funded by the drug companies, showing that, when we are feeling sad or depressed, our brains operate differently. This leads the researchers, and some mental health practitioners, to wrongly conclude that it is the brain that has caused the depression. We believe it is the other way round: that is, the brain is reacting to the depressing event, whether it involves loss or not (Read & Moncrieff, 2022). This is, after all, what the brain is supposed to do. It is the organ in our body that reacts and adjusts to the environment, helping us adapt to a changing world. If it did not operate differently in circumstances such as bereavement and loss, it would be a cause for concern.

It is also true, however, that the longer the brain stays in its depressed state, the longer it can take for it to return to its non-depressed state, hence the temptation to try to kick-start it back to 'normality' with chemicals or electric shocks. The *DSM* approach (see Chapter 4) to the challenge of deciding when, after the death of a loved one, our sadness and lack of motivation to do everyday things is a natural grieving process and when it is a mental disorder is interesting. The *DSM* edition (*DSM-IV-TR*) (APA, 2000) that preceded the current one (*DSM-5*) (APA, 2013) stated that it is a natural process for the first 60 days, but thereafter it becomes a 'major depressive episode'. The psychiatrists involved in drawing this line did, at least, acknowledge that sadness after loss is normal – but only up to a point. Where would you draw the line? Clearly if you are still feeling dreadful and unable to get on with your life five years after the death of your husband, wife, mother or father, then that is a problem. What about three years? One year?

There are individual differences (again, everyone is different). There are also cultural variations – some might say two weeks would be indicative of major depression in the archetypal stiff-upper-lipped English, while for the more emotionally expressive Irish, any period less than 12 months would be considered problematic (please excuse the stereotyping). We are not trying to make light of a difficult life event – we simply want to get across the futility of setting an arbitrary cut-off point at which mourning becomes a mental illness. We never tire of repeating that people are all different and some of those differences are determined by the culture and family we grew up in, but the medical model of mental illness and psychiatric diagnoses is set on pathologising the naturally variable grieving process.

Moreover, in 2013, the authors of *DSM-5* took a huge step backwards on this issue. They got rid of the 'bereavement exclusion' period altogether. Now, mourning for a lost loved one can be diagnosed as major depressive disorder from day one!

It is our life history before the loss (including how many other losses we have suffered), combined with the response of others around us and the quality of our life outside the lost relationship (and, yes, our cultural norms) that determine how long we grieve. Such sadness is not an indicator of a mental disorder or something wrong with our genes or the neurotransmitters in our brains.

Loss comes in many shapes and sizes – we are not only talking about the death of a loved one. We all lose friendships and romantic relationships. Losses also occur all the time in less intimate areas of our lives. The loss of a job can be devastating financially and, if our self-esteem is highly determined by our work status, emotionally.

We guess that most readers will not have got through the year without suffering one or more of the following:

- the death of a loved one
- a miscarriage
- the break-up of a marriage or life-partnership
- a son or daughter leaving home
- losing your job
- being robbed or burgled
- losing money on a bad investment
- your favoured political party losing an election
- realising that a long-held dream isn't ever going to come true.

Perhaps, in a very good year, your biggest loss might be that your football team yet again fails to win the league. (It has happened to both of us every year for the past 40 years.)

Some losses are less obvious than others. One type of loss that often goes unnoticed is the loss of our hopes. The continuous failure to realise any of our aspirations can be as chronically damaging as some of the more obvious, one-off losses discussed above. Some people, the relatively well-off for instance, have a better chance of having at least some of their dreams come true. A feeling of loss can also occur when we realise that we didn't get something that most others did get (or that we persuade ourselves most others got), or that we feel we should have had. We might realise that our childhood circumstances represent a loss. A 'lost childhood' is a term familiar to us all. We usually mean that the child was not provided with the basics that we would all hope every child would enjoy, physically and emotionally, or was subjected to torments and deprivations no child should have to endure. We mention these less tangible losses to draw readers' attention to the full range of losses that should be considered when trying to figure out where our 'problems' have come from.

While it is often true that time heals, it is also important to acknowledge that some losses, like the death of a son or daughter, for instance, fall into a category of losses that may never be completely 'recovered' from. Some losses remain an important part of the rest of our lives, and it is right that they should. It does not mean there is something wrong with us, that we have a mental disorder. However, in turn, nor does it mean that we don't sometimes need help from other people – relatives, friends and even occasionally, professionals (preferably someone who, like the public, understands that being depressed after a loss makes sense).

Before offering just one or two research studies demonstrating the obvious link between loss and mental health difficulties, we should touch on one more factor: namely, that two people experiencing a similar loss, let's say of a spouse, can react quite differently. We have already mentioned other personal determining factors, such as other recent losses and the reactions of those around us. Yet another factor is what we tell ourselves about the loss. For instance, if we decide it was our fault, partly or completely, we are more likely to be more depressed, and to stay depressed for longer. If, after losing your job, you believe it was because your boss is a fool or because the economic system is rubbish, you may well feel angry. But you will probably feel less depressed than if you tell yourself that you lost your job because you are incompetent or useless and therefore deserved to be sacked.

What we tell ourselves is particularly important after the suicide of someone we love. It is almost impossible, when that happens, not to dwell on what you might have done differently – to blame yourself in some way. This is true for mental health professionals too. Some of them, especially those who work with the most distressed people, will experience suicides of people they have come to care deeply about. If you try hard enough, you will indeed find something you could have done, or not done, that might possibly have made a difference. But you will never know for certain.

The important point is that the degree to which we blame ourselves for the loss will play a part in how long it takes us to move on. We will return to this important cause of mental health problems – our thoughts and beliefs – when we consider cognitive theory in the next chapter.

It might seem unnecessary to provide research evidence to support what folk wisdom and public opinion assume – that a serious loss, or multiple losses, can play a significant role in the development of mental health problems. But since current mental health treatment is likely to pathologise grieving and prioritise medication over talking therapies or allowing time to heal us, we will mention just two of the many studies available. Again they focus on the type of problems that many psychiatrists believe are most biological and least social in origin – psychosis and 'schizophrenia'.

A British study found that 390 people with a first episode of psychosis were twice as likely as a control group to have been separated for at least a year from one of their parents before age 16, three times more likely to have had one of their parents die, and 12 times more likely to have had their mother die (Morgan et al., 2007). These findings were after controlling for parental history of mental illness, yet again casting doubt on the genetic predisposition requirement for psychosis. As is the case for child abuse, the younger the child when the loss occurs, the greater the potential long-term consequences. Among people who had lost a parent in childhood, those who were later diagnosed with 'schizophrenia' had been bereaved an average of two years earlier (at an average age of about six years old) than those in a control group. An Israeli study found that the death of, or permanent separation from, a parent was only predictive of a 'schizophrenia' diagnosis if it occurred in the first eight years of life (Read & Gumley, 2008).

Day-to-day stress

The public are also right to identify as major causes of mental health problems social and environmental stressors like life events, family problems, social, economic and financial pressures, relationship breakdown and day-to-day problems such as famiy arguments and difficulties at work. This seems so obvious that we will not waste space on research studies demonstrating that stress levels are related to just about every mental health problem in the *DSM*. It seems that some of us are more sensitive to stressors than others. While professionals and academics might quibble about whether this variation in sensitivity depends on our genes or our childhoods (we think the answer is both), we almost all agree that day-to-day stress is hugely important in determining who cracks up or gives up and who doesn't.

Conclusion

Of course, there are other causes of mental health problems. And the causes are different for each of us. They can also be different at different points in our lives, depending on what is happening around us. Academics have their own agendas and tend to research what they think are causes in the first place, probably missing other causes in the process. An example of this comes from the vitally important field of suicide research. Traditional, biologically oriented researchers investigate whether people who kill themselves have high rates of an illness called 'depression'. Researchers who are more interested in why people get so depressed tend to research factors like poverty and child abuse. Naturally, both groups find their hypotheses confirmed!

Many years ago, one of John's research students wanted to research the issue of New Zealand's high youth suicide rate. She brought no preconceptions or specific hypotheses; she simply asked several hundred New Zealanders aged 18–24 years (the age bracket at highest risk) why they thought the rate was so high. The most commonly cited cause of suicide was pressure to conform and perform, followed by financial worries, abuse and neglect, problems with alcohol or drugs, and boredom. Mental illness was cited by only 1%. Many people may be surprised that pressure to conform and perform and boredom might be such major contributors.

Having discussed a rather long list of possible causes, we move on in the next chapter to discuss *how* these various factors lead to mental health problems.[3]

---

[3]. You can find recent presentations of John's views about psychosis and other mental health problems at www.madinamerica.com/2019/05/an-interview-with-dr-john-read and www.youtube.com/watch?v=0aSSB1tctxY

Chapter 7
Psychological theories: how events operate on us to create problems

We all have our preferred ways of understanding ourselves and other people, although we may not all be bold enough to turn them into formal theories, as some psychologists do. Do you think mental health problems come about largely because some people tell themselves negative things about themselves? Or do you prefer to focus on the types of relationships we develop early in life that we then repeat over and over again? Maybe you think that severe distress is an understandable, if sometimes extreme, coping reaction to distressing life events and that, if health-promoting conditions prevail, we have the capacity to recover ourselves? Perhaps you like the idea that we learn unhelpful ways of behaving from having them reinforced when we were younger? Or do you follow the path of unconscious desires and conflicts?

There are many psychological theories about how human beings develop their patterns of behaving, thinking and feeling. These are called 'personality theories', 'developmental theories' or 'psychological models'. They try to explain both 'normal' and 'abnormal' ways of interacting with the world – or, as Pete has previously written:

> the study of personality is the study of human psychological structure – how people are put together, how they work and… how they fall apart. (Sanders, 2006a, p.16)

Each of the many theories has different explanations of the causes of mental health problems and carries their ideas through to form the bases of different types of psychological treatments. So a psychodynamic/psychoanalytic therapist will follow the theories developed by Sigmund Freud and his followers, a humanistic person-centred therapist will base their ideas and practice on the work of Carl Rogers, while a cognitive therapist will see value in and follow the theories and techniques of Aaron Beck and his followers.

Understanding a little about the six theories summarised here may help you think through how psychological problems start and sometimes develop into ongoing, life-affecting patterns. It may also help you understand how therapy can help clients figure out what is currently getting in the way of overcoming (or accepting) them. This knowledge may also help you understand what psychologists, counsellors or psychotherapists think and what they are trying to do to help their patients or clients. However, we would always suggest that a good mental health professional should explain their theory or model to their clients at the outset. If they don't – we should ask them.

You will already lean towards certain explanations according to your family culture, religious beliefs, education and experiences in life – including, most importantly, your experiences of emotional distress. The ideas and language we use when thinking and talking about psychological distress are a clue to how we might favour different theories. We will see as we go along how, over the years, the language of psychological theories has crept into our everyday thinking. We suggest that, after considering all the theories summarised here, you take what makes sense to you and 'disregard the rest'.

Psychoanalysis

Before we get into introducing the ideas of Sigmund Freud (1856–1939), we need to explain something about the current use of terminology. 'Psychoanalysis' usually refers to a rather strict belief in the original teachings of Sigmund Freud – who, understandably, is revered by some in the mental health world (Freud et al., 1953–74). 'Psychodynamic' is a broader term that includes psychoanalysis and all the many ideas that have built upon, and branched out from, Freud's original theories. Over time, Freud, and most other major psychological theorists, revised and developed their ideas, which were later further revised and developed by their students and followers.

Psychodynamic theories can be quite complicated. So, if you try reading psychodynamic theorists' original writings and you don't get it, don't think you need to keep at it until it sinks in – maybe it's just not for you. Move on until you find something that makes sense. Psychodynamic (and humanistic) thinkers include factors that are hard to measure – in the case of psychodynamic theories, things like the unconscious, dreams and so on. They are often criticised by more hard-nosed psychologists for not being 'scientific'. Maybe you have your own thoughts on how scientific psychology should be. One problem is that there are multiple views about what exactly constitutes science, and whether the type of scientific methodology used to understand rocks or classify plants is the best approach to understanding human beings. Unfortunately we don't have the space to discuss those issues here. We'll confine ourselves to the content of the theories and leave you to make up your own mind.

Human development

Freud thought that human adult personality is the result of a few fundamental elements of humanness developed into a unique person by early experiences. He reasoned that all humans go through broadly the same set of life experiences as they develop into adults. Namely, we all have to be weaned onto solid food; we all have to learn to control our bowels; we all have to develop our sexuality, and we all have to become capable of separate existence from our parents or primary caregivers. These milestones of human development are achieved in all cultures, but in each culture (and, of course, each family within that culture) by slightly different means. Each culture and each family has different rituals and practices to achieve these transitions.

Without going into detail, Freud and his followers thought that how these landmark events are handled by each family leads to differences between us in terms of how we react to the world. For example, the sort of things that we get anxious about, the ways we seek comfort, and how much we want to control our surroundings, are all thought to be due to the way these important, essential life stages were conducted in our early years, from overly controlling to overly permissive parenting.

As we proceed through these stages of development, our essential humanness is unfolding. The interaction between the two (developmental transitions and unfolding essential humanness) weaves our personality into three parts. These three parts are:

- *The id* – this is the part of the personality that we are born with. Freud described the id as a seething cauldron of instincts and desires that seek gratification at all costs. Id processes are unconscious. We are not only unaware of them; they are so primitive and survival-oriented that they are almost dangerous and chaotic. They are ultimately pleasure- and comfort-seeking. The id has no values, morals or concept of right and wrong. Its workings are most clearly seen in the behaviour of a new-born baby. Freud called the inborn energy of the id the life energy or libido. He believed that it was largely sexual in nature.

- *The super-ego* – this is the conscience – the internalised, rule-enforcing parent part of the personality. Freud believed that the super-ego is formed when the child identifies with the same-sex parent, changing 'You mustn't do this' to 'I mustn't do this', and so internalising rules, morals, notions of right and wrong, gender roles and so on. The development of the super-ego is basically a learning process. The strength of the super-ego is explained by the fact that it develops at a very early age (around five years old), when young children are very vulnerable and impressionable. It is in permanent conflict with the gratification-seeking, rule-breaking id.

- *The ego* – the ego develops through childhood, first as a mediator between the chaotic id and the outside world. The ego works out the consequences of behaviour aimed at satisfying the id and applies reality, and the brakes, to the impulses of the id. Later, the ego has to appease the demands of the super-ego, so its task becomes a delicate balancing act. The ego is only fully developed at maturity. A properly adjusted adult is governed by the ego, balancing the 'I want it now!' demands of the id against the 'You mustn't do this, you naughty child!' admonishments of the super-ego.

Freud proposed that there were three domains of mental life: the conscious domain, the pre-conscious domain and the unconscious domain. We might picture these domains stacked on top of each other, with the unconscious at the bottom, inaccessible, hidden and unknown. The pre-conscious is in the middle, acting as a half-way house, and the conscious is on top, known, available and present as the mediator of everyday living.

The unconscious is the domain of the taboo id impulses that are the source of the very life of the organism, being concerned with survival, sex, comfort and bodily functions. These primitive, animalistic impulses, argued Freud, must be kept hidden from our awareness, confined to the unconscious domain, denied admission to the conscious in their raw, often offensive form. It is by keeping these impulses 'in their proper place' that a healthy dynamic equilibrium is maintained by the ego. There is, however, a problem. As well as being taboo, the id energy is also life-giving and life-sustaining; it is the source of our creative energy and we need these impulses in order to live a fulfilling life.

The ego defends the conscious mind against raw id impulses by creating a barrier through which they can only gain admission by various roundabout ways, becoming acceptable in the process. This re-routing takes the form of what are called ego defences or defence mechanisms. Since id energy must gain expression somehow, we are all using defence mechanisms all of the time.

Ego defences can be successful, allowing expression of the forbidden impulse in a way that gives the id satisfaction; or they can be unsuccessful, simply preventing expression and causing the impulse to re-present itself over and over again, each time demanding satisfaction. Unsuccessful ego defence leaves undischarged energy in the system, which must go somewhere, and so is eventually expressed as anxiety. Defence mechanisms are not necessarily pathological; they serve, for all of us, the invaluable function of keeping undesirable drives, feelings and memories out of awareness. Without defence mechanisms, we would be completely unable to get on with our day-to-day lives. Yet Freud believed that some were healthier than others.

Successful ego-defence is called sublimation and is achieved by deflecting the impulse into an acceptable activity, so:

- the impulse to be aggressive is satisfied by playing competitive sport
- the desire to handle faeces becomes an interest in pottery.

There are lots of less successful ego defences – including, for example:

- *Repression*, which is the process of keeping taboo impulses and any related ideas out of consciousness, so that we are completely unaware of them. To be effective, the process itself has to be unconscious too.

- *Reaction-formation*, which is the formation of feelings in the conscious that are the opposite of the unconscious id impulses. Examples are love becoming hate (most teenagers will understand this!), and over-moralising and exaggerated disgust as reactions against sexuality.

- *Projection*, which is the attribution of our own taboo impulses to others. So 'I hate him', which is unacceptable because I like to think of myself as a kind person or because I am scared I will kill the bastard, becomes 'He hates me'. When it is combined with reaction-formation, we can see how a chain of events develops: 'I love him' becomes 'I hate him' (via reaction-formation), which in turn becomes 'He hates me' (via projection). Since the original taboo impulses are unconscious and therefore not known to us, this chain of events is out of our awareness and the first we know is that we get a strong notion that a new acquaintance dislikes us from the off. So, a common form of projection is when self-hatred (which is unacceptable) is projected onto the other person as 'You don't like me,' or, 'You hate me'.

- *Turning feelings against self* might seem to be an idea in conflict with projection, but it is yet another way of denying an unacceptable impulse. This time, if I have aggressive feelings towards someone I love (an unacceptable impulse), I can turn them back on myself. This can lead to self-doubt, self-loathing, depression and, in extreme cases, self-harm and suicide.

Dreams

You can't really talk about psychoanalysis without discussing dreams. One of Freud's most famous books is *The Interpretation of Dreams*, first published in 1899. A more recent illustrated edition (Freud, 2010) is particularly beautiful, and includes fascinating commentary by Freud's famous 'critical friend' Jeffrey Masson (see below). Freud called dreams 'the royal road to the unconscious'. While the usually vigilant ego is having a rest, the id is free to run rampant. Like 'Freudian slips' (for example, 'Hello. I don't believe we've been properly seduced'), dreams can help us discover our deeper desires and fears, however surprising or unflattering they may be. If you want to use your own dreams to help you understand yourself, do not buy a dream dictionary that tells you that, for instance, all trains represent penises and all tunnels are vaginas. Freud was very clear that we develop our own symbols. Instead, buy a notebook and (if you can catch your dreams first thing when you wake – which is the hard part because the ego wakes up pretty fast and puts the lid back on), jot down as much of them as you can remember. After a few weeks, read through your notes and see what comes to you, what patterns emerge. But remember that not all dreams are deep and meaningful. Some are just a repeating of the mundane events of the day before.

Freud's disciples

Freud's ideas were spread widely by his students and followers, to the extent that hundreds of thousands of people all over the world now practise what Freud preached. The better-known of them are those who have dissented to some extent and established their own variations. We offer just a few examples here. Carl Jung (1875–1961) was one of the first to break ranks, with his emphasis on the spiritual world, his belief in a collective unconscious shared by all of us, and his ideas about us all being made up of opposite and competing parts, like the archetypal female – Jung called it the 'anima' – and male, or 'animus'. *Man and his Symbols,* one of Jung's last works, written in 1961, is also published in a beautifully illustrated edition (Jung, 1961/1997).

Harry Stack Sullivan (his main work, *The Interpersonal Theory of Psychiatry*, was published in 1953) and Frieda Fromm-Reichman (*Psychoanalysis and Psychosis* (1989)) developed Freud's understanding of psychosis as a response to what had happened to people and how that led them to distort their world. Joanna Greenberg's account of being in therapy with Fromm-Reichman following a psychotic breakdown, *I Never Promised You a Rose Garden*, is a riveting read (Greenberg, 1964).

Erich Fromm (1900–1980) challenged some of the sexist aspects of Freud's thinking (women do not really envy penises or want to have sex with their father!) and built on Freud's ideas to address social and political phenomenon (Fromm, 1956, 2002). He reframed our central conflict thus:

> It is the paradox of human existence that man must simultaneously seek for closeness and for independence; for oneness with others and at the same time for the preservation of his uniqueness and particularity... the answer to this paradox – and to the moral problems of man – is productiveness. (Fromm, 2003)

Sándor Ferenczi seemed destined to become Freud's chosen successor until he insisted that Freud had been correct, early in his career, to point out that most of his female patients had been sexually abused as children. Freud had soon retracted this early belief that many of his clients had been sexually abused and replaced it with the (very different) idea that children fantasise about having sex with their parents. More recently, the psychoanalyst Jeffrey Masson similarly didn't think it was a good idea to base a whole school of thought on the idea that, if someone tells you they were abused as a child, you should assume it is just a fantasy. He discovered in Freud's unpublished letters evidence that Freud never really stopped believing in sexual abuse as a primary cause of mental health problems and that he had been pressured into retracting his claim by his peers and colleagues. Masson offers us a gripping account of one of the most important debates of the 20th century in his wonderful book *The Assault on Truth* (1984).

We have no way of knowing whether the psychodynamic approach – or any of the other theories that follow – will be of any use to you in your thinking about the causes of your difficulties in life or those of your loved ones or clients. We do know that some of the basic ideas of psychoanalytic theory make sense to, and are accepted by, millions of people around the world. Many of Freud's central ideas – like dream interpretation and Freudian slips – have become part of popular culture. And he was, perhaps surprisingly, accepting of homosexuality, which he regarded as simply a variation of sexual expression and not something to be treated by psychoanalysis. Some people find some psychoanalytic ideas over-complicated and hard to grasp, and therefore rather irritating or even nonsensical. It is perhaps best to start with a brief introductory text (Appignanesi & Zarate, 2003; Storr, 2001).

Attachment theory

British psychiatrist John Bowlby (1907–1990) was originally a psychoanalyst but became interested in Konrad Lorenz's research into how young chicks, and other creatures, become 'imprinted' on or attached to – and follow around – the first available adult (of any species, or indeed an inanimate object if it is in the right place at the right time). Bowlby's seminal work, *Attachment and Loss*, published in three volumes, in 1969, 1973 and 1980, presented the findings from his research on homeless and orphaned children in post-war Europe that he conducted for the World Health Organization. It is still available and is the basis for modern-day attachment theory. Early separation from parents was a major problem in Britain during World War II, because of the deaths of so many men in active service and of whole families in the bombing of civilian urban centres, and also prolonged separation due to the evacuation of children from cities.

Another of his books, *Child Care and the Growth of Love* (1951), influenced the provision of care for orphaned children throughout the developed world. His work is still instructive reading for anyone interested in the causes of mental health problems.

Bowlby's attachment theory argues that a baby's first relationship with an adult, their primary caregiver(s) (usually, but not always, the mother), is hugely important in how we relate to others as adults. He argued that the quality of that first relationship (or relationships) largely determines how we relate to other people when we are adults. At a very young age, we develop 'internal models' of what we expect relationships to be like and behave accordingly.

American researcher Mary Ainsworth (1913–1999) used Bowlby's theory in her famous 'Strange Situation' experiment. She observed how toddlers react when their mum leaves them alone in a room and when she returns. She identified three 'attachment styles'. The first (shown by about 70% of the children) she called 'secure attachment'. These children were a little upset when mum left but greeted her when she came back and were easily comforted. About 20% of the children, those with 'avoidant attachment', took little notice when mum left and shunned her when she returned. The third group (about 10%) became very disturbed when mum left, and when she came back alternated between reaching to be picked up and angrily squirming to be put down. Ainsworth called this 'ambivalent attachment' (Ainsworth & Bell, 1970).

Subsequent research has shown that these attachment styles, learned very early in life, can indeed influence our relationships as adults (Cervone & Pervin, 2008, pp.147–155). Unsurprisingly, those of us with a secure attachment style tend to find it fairly easy to make friends and to trust them. Those of us who learned an avoidant style find it difficult to depend on and trust others, and often keep a safe emotional distance that other people can find difficult. Those who developed an ambivalent attachment style when they were little may yearn to have a very close (almost merged) relationship with someone but can become obsessively worried about whether they love them as much in return and fearful that they will leave them. This, understandably, tends to scare other people away, which can become a self-fulfilling prophecy.

More recent work on attachment styles has developed the theory to offer 'universal truths' about the effects of impaired attachment. In particular, psychodynamic psychologist Peter Fonagy has linked adult mental health to attachment styles, while embracing neuropsychology (Fonagy et al., 2004). He has explored in great detail the different types of attachment, arguing that stable adult mental health requires the attachment figure (usually the mother) to have provided a relationship that is both contained (safe) and regulated. If the parent is themselves beset by problems, ranging from drug dependency through to poverty, their ability to provide the right sort of attachment relationship is compromised.

Be careful not to put yourself, or your parents or carers, too rigidly in one of these categories – they are not 'boxes', they are a spectrum along which we may be positioned at different points in our lives, rather than a permanent state. It remains the case, though, that these theories about particular styles of attachment can sometimes be useful when trying to understand a person's current relational difficulties and how they emerged. If you conclude that your parents or early caregivers did not help you develop a secure attachment style, just remember that they had childhoods and parents too!

Learning theories

Learning theories were at the centre of the emerging field of behaviourism in the early 20th century. Learning theories are not concerned with early relationships with our mums or our dreams or unconscious fears and desires. The founders of behaviourism were, in their determination to make psychology scientific, only interested in what could be reliably measured. The behavioural approaches, more than any other theory up to that point, used academic psychology as their starting point. Much of modern psychology owes a great deal to the work of early behaviourists. Behaviourism grew to dominate American psychology by the middle of the century. J.B. Watson (1878–1958) and B.F. Skinner (1904–1990), working separately and on different learning processes, founded the movement that Skinner hoped would set humans free from the shackles of their existence by developing a technology of change and making it available to everyone – science to set everyone free (Skinner, 1948).

The basic principles of behaviourism are:

- apparently complex behaviour is a collection of more simple elements that can be understood in terms of basic learning principles
- whatever has been learned can be unlearned and modified through the application of learning principles.

Careful unravelling the 'what has been learned' and 'how it was learned' is the key to understanding learning that has been unhelpful or has led to distressing outcomes or symptoms. Once understood, it can be unlearned and more positive behaviour learned in its place.

There are two ways in which a new pattern of behaviour can be acquired – two types of learning. They are called classical conditioning and operant conditioning (Cash, 2021; Cromby et al., 2013a).

Classical conditioning

Classical conditioning is a type of stimulus-response relationship where a stimulus becomes associated with a reflex response. Ivan Pavlov, the famous Russian physiologist, stumbled on the procedure about 100 years ago, while studying the salivary reflex. He noticed that, if a dog was fed from the same bowl by the same lab technician repeatedly, the dog would start to salivate at the sight of the bowl alone and even at the sight of the lab technician. Note that salivation is a reflex that happens in anticipation of food to prepare for its digestion. Thousands of experiments followed, using the same principle: that a (previously) 'neutral' stimulus (the sight of the lab technician) can produce a 'conditioned response' (salivation) through its association with a stimulus (food) that automatically produces the same response. It has provided a useful model to help us understand other such seemingly reflex responses, such as phobias.

John B. Watson, with his colleague Rosalie Rayner, conducted the famous 'Little Albert' experiment – one that would certainly not get past the ethics committee today. They presented a small boy, called Albert, with a white rat (which had previously attracted Albert's interest), while simultaneously making a loud noise by striking a metal bar with a hammer just behind Albert's head. He was frightened by the noise and began to associate the noise with the presence of the white rat. After a few such 'pairings' (of the rat and the loud noise), Albert cried every time the rat was brought near him. This demonstrated that a fear reflex could be learned and associated with a neutral object – which explained how we can become fearful of seemingly 'neutral' objects, animals or situations.

Several classical conditioning experiments demonstrated the important idea of 'generalisation', whereby we can become fearful of things because they are similar to the stimulus we have become frightened of. Soldiers returning from active duty often find that they are panicked by any loud noise that is similar to their frightening battlefield experiences. Similarly, people who have been abused as kids often feel fearful in the presence of someone who resembles the abuser. If other people don't know about our life histories, we can look pretty mad if we 'over-react' (have a 'conditioned emotional reaction') to a car backfiring or to a man with a moustache entering the room.

Operant conditioning

Operant conditioning is fundamentally different in that it describes the way voluntary behaviours (as opposed to reflexes) become associated with stimuli. It describes the process by which behaviours are 'shaped' by whether they are reinforced (rewarded) or not. The basic idea is that we are more likely to repeat a behaviour if something good happens immediately after, every time (or most times) we do it. B.F. Skinner conducted a series of pioneering experiments where he automated the whole process of training rats and pigeons to do a range of things in his 'Skinner box' by giving them food pellets as rewards immediately afterwards.

Skinner had no time for colleagues who wanted to use diagnoses or label people 'normal' or 'abnormal', 'sane' or 'crazy'. He preferred to understand our differences in terms of our personal history of what had, and had not, been reinforced. In very simplistic terms, a shy person with great difficulty making friends would be understood as not having had many social skills reinforced (they would have a 'behavioural deficit'), while someone who does 'bad' or 'mad' things will have learned those behaviours by being rewarded for them somewhere along the line. When we say 'learned', we must realise that life presents us with many situations that resemble a Skinner box. If a person gains relief from voices in their head by shouting back at them, you can see how behaviour perceived by others as 'mad' might be learned. If we take the trouble to discover a person's history, we might understand their 'strange' behaviour. Other psychological models might help us understand why they hear voices in the first place.

All parents are using 'operant conditioning' every time they praise their children for being helpful or polite, perhaps without realising there is a scientific name for it. Most people instinctively recognise the value of rewarding certain behaviours and ignoring the behaviours you don't want. It works. It's important to note that Skinner and others clearly demonstrated that the way to get rid of unwanted behaviour is a process of 'extinction' or lack of reinforcement, not punishment. The application of aversive stimuli – punishment, in ordinary language – does not extinguish unwanted behaviour. It only suppresses it until the punishment stops. People who advocate the 'carrot and stick' approach have only got it half right.

The carrot works but the stick doesn't

Operant conditioning might apply to the causes of mental health problems. For example:

- *Depression* can be thought of as a general lack of reinforcement. For human beings, a reinforcement is, by definition, something that makes us feel good. If nothing good happens to us for a long period of time, no matter what we try to do, we start doing less and less. The less we do, the fewer rewards we receive and the more depressed we get. So we can get into a downward spiral of doing less and less and feeling worse and worse. This suggests that the cure for this is to force ourselves (perhaps with the help of a friend) to do something, anything, however trivial, that makes us feel good. Gradually, and with a lot of effort at first, we can start to remember what it is like to feel good (even for a couple of minutes), and we then have a little more energy to do a little more, which makes us feel a little better, and thus we can replace the downward spiral with an upwards one. This, however, takes more effort than staying depressed or drowning our sorrows in bottles of pills, alcohol or street drugs.

- *Gambling addiction* is easily understood once we understand that certain 'schedules of reinforcement' are particularly hard to 'extinguish'. Skinner showed that, after a behaviour has become established through repeated reinforcement, it can be 'extinguished' by removing the reward. After a few repetitions of pressing the bar and no food pellet arriving, the rat stops pressing. However, if the original learning had involved a random schedule of reinforcement (the relationship between pressing the bar and whether the food pellet arrives), where it's impossible to predict when the food will arrive (i.e. every so often, with no pattern to it), then the bar-pressing behaviour becomes extremely difficult to extinguish. This is the type of reinforcement schedule programmed into slot and gaming machines and the responses (putting the money in and pulling the handle) are very difficult to stop – just one more pull, the next one might be the one!

So, learning theory places great emphasis on our environment – on the events and people that shape our behaviour. We are all reinforcing, ignoring or punishing one another all the time. It is how we get what we want from one another and negotiate the world. It could be that some of us have had things that make us uncomfortable or distressed reinforced too often or haven't had the things that help us feel joyful and fulfilled reinforced enough.

Social learning theory

Social learning theory is most associated with Albert Bandura (1925–2021). Of the many ideas that come under this general heading, we have chosen two that we think might be particularly helpful when trying to understand the causes of our emotional difficulties: observational learning, and self-reinforcement, both of which are examples of 'social learning theory' (Bandura, 1977).

Observational learning is just a fancy term for copying other people. You don't need to be a psychologist to know that a lot of how we behave or feel is simply the result of imitating others – often automatically, without knowing we are doing it. It could originate from the fact that we humans, like many other animals, are social creatures and must learn to fit in with what goes on around us.

Any parent of a teenager understands just how powerful an influence peer pressure can be, as we feel our parental influence beginning to fade away. However, imitation starts much earlier than that. As children, we all copy mum and dad, or older brothers and sisters, then school friends, and even teachers, and so on. Observational learning is essentially copying what we have seen without it actually being reinforced. We just do it because we have seen it. Other experiments have found the perhaps equally obvious fact that we are particularly likely to copy certain types of people, especially powerful people, those we like or respect and those we want to be like. We are all familiar with the term 'role model'; it's just that young people refuse to choose the right ones!

So, when trying to understand how you respond when life throws hard stuff at you, have a think about how mum and dad (or whoever your earliest 'role model' was) dealt with hard stuff. When you do this, it becomes obvious why it is silly to assume that, just because depression or psychosis or anxiety or whatever 'runs in families', the best way to understand that is to start looking at genes. Our patterns of how we respond when bad things happen to us (or when good things don't) often go back several generations. Where do you think your dad learned to be the way he was? Who did he copy?

Bandura conducted a famous experiment in which children observed an adult behaving violently towards a child-sized, skittle-like doll that bounced back upright when hit or kicked. When the children were allowed back in the playroom, they imitated the adult's violent behaviour. This became known as 'vicarious learning', 'observational learning' or 'modelling'. The interesting feature was that the young children were not actively rewarded for copying the adult's behaviour; they just seemed to do it naturally. This finding from Bandura leads to the social learning theory idea that, rather than just being passive victims of reinforcements in our early childhoods, we continually set ourselves goals and can reinforce or punish ourselves for our progress, or lack thereof, towards those goals. While psychoanalysis and behaviourism may feel good as explanations because we are less responsible for the messes we get into, the social learning theory notion is a bit more challenging as we have to accept more responsibility. The idea is that we can, to a large extent, set our own compass and help ourselves move in our chosen direction by praising ourselves for any progress. This 'self-talk' idea overlaps with cognitive theory, which we will cover next.

Cognitive theory

When behaviourism was at its height, psychologists were not too interested in thoughts. Measuring what goes on in the 'black box' of our own skulls was extremely difficult (if not heresy), and so didn't pass muster as real 'science'. Cognitive psychology (the study of thought processes) did thrive during and after World War II, but mainly as a way of helping us understand the sort of mistakes people made when looking at radar screens or when having to make a decision after being on duty for 48 hours without a break. It wasn't until the 1960s that Aaron Beck (1921–2021) pressed cognitive theory into practice as a model for psychological distress. Albert Ellis (1913–2007), originator of rational emotive behaviour therapy, was another pioneer of this approach, for which he developed detailed theory and practice protocols (Cromby et al., 2013a; Hills & Pake, 2016).

When first encountering cognitive therapy, some people find the idea of changing people's thoughts a bit disrespectful, possibly intrusive or, in extreme cases, a sort of mind control. However, like so many things pressed into practice to help someone who is desperate, in the hands of a good, sensitive practitioner, many patients and clients experience it as informative, helpful and even liberating.

The basic model is wonderfully simple. Usually, when a depressing thing happens, we feel depressed. What has caused the feeling? Obviously, the depressing event. Not necessarily, argue the cognitive theorists. Their evidence is that, faced with the same event, not all of us will be equally depressed, and some of us won't be the slightest bit bothered. What makes the difference? What we tell ourselves about the event, or about ourselves. This is the A-B-C model, where A is the event, C is the feeling that follows the event, and B – the all-important factor – is our thoughts about the event or ourselves.

The following example might help explain the process. (John has used it for 20 years in his undergraduate lectures.) After weeks of trying to get up the courage, you finally ask someone you have long had your eye on out on a date. To your astonishment, they agree. You arrange to meet outside a cinema. The big day arrives. You arrive on time, and you wait, and wait and… you go home, feeling very down. Wouldn't everyone feel the same? The answer is no. It depends on many things – such as how many times this has happened before. But a major determinant is that little voice inside you trying to make sense of it all. You can tell yourself it's because you are ugly, because you are somehow just unlovable. You can tell yourself you'll never have a girlfriend or boyfriend. The list of ways to put yourself down is endless. Or you could assume there was a plausible reason why the other person didn't show – maybe something unexpected happened to interrupt their plans. Or you could be a bit grandiose and convince yourself that anyone who didn't realise that you were the best catch around wasn't worth bothering with!

The thing is, most of us have one or two 'negative self-statements' we use to bash ourselves over the heads with whenever something goes wrong. They are different for each of us, but whichever ones we are burdened with, they are like a little close-looped audiotape lurking just below the surface of consciousness waiting to be triggered by something, anything, bad happening. We have our ready-made explanation.

John's main one used to be (and on a bad day still is) that he is stupid, dumb, unintelligent. It played itself in different keys – including 'If you weren't so thick you would have known that would happen' – but the melody was always the same. Cognitive therapy is designed to help us catch these thoughts. This is not easy because they happen automatically and often without awareness, which is why a cognitive therapist will ask you to keep a thought diary. If you can catch your own particular ways of putting yourself down, the next step is to start the work of replacing them with something a little more helpful and realistic. Not 'I am Albert Einstein', but perhaps 'I am sometimes quite clever at some things'.

But this book is about causes not treatments. Readers wanting an honest evaluation of psychological treatments could read the chapter on 'Interventions' in John Cromby, Dave Harper and Paula Reavey's book *Psychology, Mental Health and Distress* (2013e) (a second edition is due to be published in 2023).

Cognitive theory suggests that mental health problems are caused by our inaccurate and negative thoughts about ourselves, about the world, about the future and so on. That is an idea that most readers will be able to identify with. But without exploring where the ideas came from in the first place, you can end up being even more hard on yourself, with statements like, 'Oh my god, not only am I depressed, obsessive, alcoholic, anxious or whatever – I am also one of those people who has negative self-statements!'

To understand the causes of mental health problems from a cognitive perspective, you need to try to discover where the 'cognitions' came from. How, for instance, did someone like John

– who was almost always top of his class – end up telling himself he was stupid? Well, like you, he learned his own special way of putting himself down early in life. Many people discover that the negative self-talk, the words going round in circles in their heads waiting to be released by some unfortunate incident, are the words of a teacher or parent or someone else important to them in some way, who, perhaps in a moment of anger (or several moments of anger), said something about you that wasn't very nice. And it got stuck there.

Cognitive therapy practitioners would want us to explain that cognitive therapy is much more complicated than how we have described it here, but we don't have the space here to do complete justice to any of the theories we are summarising. Nevertheless, we will mention just one or two of the complexities.

First, it isn't just what we think that matters; *how* we think can be important too. We tend to develop patterns of types of thinking and some of these can cause us problems. Some examples include:

- *selective abstraction* – focusing only on the negative aspects of a situation, such as the one thing you forgot to do today, rather than all the things you did remember to do
- *overgeneralisation* – drawing big conclusions on the basis of a single, small event, such as assuming that, because you were late for work today, you are an incompetent or unvalued worker
- *magnification and minimisation* – exaggerating bad things about ourselves while downplaying the positives
- *all-or-nothing thinking* – seeing events or people (including ourselves) as either all bad or all good, such as putting people into our 'good box' or 'bad box' within a few seconds of meeting them (or without having met them at all)
- *personalisation* – assuming that we are always responsible for other people's feeling: for instance, believing that, just because your partner is upset, you must have done something wrong (maybe you did but try asking them).

So, when a bad thing happens, we have some choices about what we tell ourselves. There are at least three dimensions to the 'attributions' we make about a bad event. These are internal-external, global–specific and permanent–temporary. If John's students want to feel really depressed the next time they get a bad grade from him, they should tell themselves:

1. that the grade was caused by something about themselves (internal) – being a bit thick will do
2. that this is a global phenomenon – they are thick at everything not just psychology, and
3. this is permanent – they have been, and always will be, thick.

Alternatively they could brighten up their day a bit by going external – 'Professor Read set an unfair exam'; specific – 'Other lecturers don't do that', and temporary – 'Even though this one was unfair, Professor Read's exams are usually fair, so this won't happen again.'

There are two potential problems in looking at things this way. First, there is a risk of blaming yourself for blaming yourself if you don't figure out where the blaming started. And second, sometimes life really is depressing. Sometimes it isn't what we tell ourselves about an event; it really is the event itself (or a series of events) that is the cause of our problems. So, we have to be careful that we don't go to the other extreme of looking at everything through rose-tinted glasses and denying that there is some pretty awful stuff happening sometimes, to ourselves and to those around us, and in the world generally. Beware the folk who try to sell you the idea that all problems can be solved by the wonders of positive thinking. In fact, there are a few studies that show that, when we are depressed, we actually see some aspects of the world (including how others judge us) more accurately than people who are not depressed (Alloy & Abramson, 1979; Haaga & Beck, 1995)! Having said that, many have found this cognitive approach to be really good when it comes to figuring out why we don't like ourselves as much as we should.

Humanistic theory

Abraham Maslow (1908–1970) is often cited as the founder of humanistic psychology. He was more interested in what makes us healthy or 'self-actualized' than what causes our mental health problems. As with the other approaches, it's difficult to summarise humanistic psychology in a page or two. In the case of humanistic psychology, this is because there are so many different approaches beneath its umbrella. The ideas were developed in the mid-20th century based on the contemporary philosophies of existentialism and phenomenology, and focusing on the prime human qualities of hope, love, creativity and the central importance of lived experience.

Existentialism is a philosophical approach with a very wide variety of thought, some of it contradicting other parts. Its key themes are the focus on lived experience, freedom and the consequent task of living one's life under one's own responsibility. Philosopher Søren Kierkegaard is now regarded as the 'father of existentialism'. Phenomenology is a philosophical approach to understanding and psychology where 'truth' or 'knowledge' comes from the perceptual field of the individual rather than from an external authority. It is based on the work of philosopher Edmund Husserl. Wikipedia is as good a place to start as any to discover more about philosophers and schools of philosophy.

Person-centred therapy

Maslow's ideas did not translate directly into a therapeutic approach, but American psychologist Carl Rogers (1902–1982) developed a theory of distress and a therapeutic method that has influenced psychology worldwide. Some of Rogers' ideas are, like Freud's, so influential that they have been incorporated into psychological therapies and are now practically taken as read and have become a sort of therapeutic common sense.

The name of Rogers' approach changed over the years, and the way this happened says something about both the man and the approach. In the late 1930s and throughout the 1940s, Rogers developed his approach from his experiences of working with patients, initially with 'problem children'. Two key principles in his early work were: i) to rely on the individual's own tendency towards growth (getting better), and ii) not to interfere too much in this or 'play the expert'. He started to call this method 'non-directive therapy', to emphasise the importance of acknowledging the idea that, if supported appropriately, people could find solutions to their own problems.

By 1951, Rogers was calling the approach 'client-centred therapy', to give more emphasis to the notion that the 'client' (rather than the medical term 'patient') was the expert in their own lives and that the therapist was in their service. Soon he changed the name one final time to 'person-centred therapy', to address even more of the power imbalance between the person wanting help and the person offering help as a companion. He was against 'expertism' and was convinced that people really could grow positively through distress if provided with the right conditions.

Carl Rogers proposed six conditions that, if present in a relationship, are 'necessary and sufficient' for therapeutic change. The conditions are: i) that the two people are in psychological contact; ii) that one identifies themselves as the client; iii) that the other identifies as the therapist; iv) the therapist must be non-judgemental and warm; v) the therapist must try to understand the client (be empathic), and vi) the client must experience these qualities in the therapist. You can find out more about Carl Rogers and person-centred therapy in Pete's highly popular and accessible book *The Person-Centred Counselling Primer* (Sanders, 2006a).

The causes of distress

It is easy to oversimplify Rogers' theory. It does have a very 'common-sense' feel to it and at the same time has several components that set it against almost all other theories and many accepted practices in mental health services. In a nutshell, Rogers stated that human infants (and adults, for that matter) need unconditional acceptance in order to grow (and maintain) a healthy self-structure. Every time they are offered conditional love (i.e. they will receive it if they behave in a certain way), they build up a set of ideas about themselves that is based not on their own experiences but on the values and judgements of others. Here Rogers is talking about a very wide range of things from, for example, sexuality ('You will only be loved and accepted if you are straight') through to expression of thoughts and feelings ('You will only be loved if you keep quiet about the abuse you are suffering'). Note also that this withholding of love can be unspoken and very subtle, or quite brutal.

This results in an 'imported' self-structure that starts to operate separately from the person's natural ability to experience the world for themselves, and when these two elements are in conflict, Rogers called this 'incongruence'. If a person has a lot of imported material (rather than that based on self-evaluated experience), they experience more and more unpleasant conflict between these two parts of themselves as they go about their everyday life in the world. It is easy to see how these internalised judgemental (or self-sustaining) elements can become experienced as 'voices'.

Some experiences will be congruent in that they 'fit' the person's view of themselves ('I am gay and being attracted to other men feels good') but many will not fit and are experienced as a threat to the whole of the self-structure ('I have these feelings that are wrong – I am bad and unlovable'). Since incongruent experiences suggest that either the experience or the self-structure is 'wrong', something has to give. Either the person denies or distorts the experience (to get rid of the incongruence), or they suffer from anxiety (anything from a relentless niggling discomfort to a panic attack), which in turn is an experience that may not fit with their image of themselves ('I'm a positive person, not someone who feels afraid all the time').

The more your personality is determined by the judgemental influence of others, the greater the discrepancy between your experiences and your self-image will be. The more discrepancy there is, the more threatened your self-structure will be. We naturally fortify our wobbly self-structure by making it more solid and rigid (ironically, by trying to support the elements within it that are causing the problem in the first place). A healthy self-structure needs to be flexible, since life unfolds in unexpected ways, and we must respond creatively, not with the same old rigid patterns.

If threatened enough (e.g. by our attempts to deny or distort past abuse, or defend against trauma, loss or unremitting stress), the brittle self-structure will eventually break, resulting in loss of identity and/or chaotic thinking and feeling.

Since the fault lines in the self-structure were caused initially by judgemental, conditional love, 'treatment' is intended to offer a therapeutic relationship 'involving primarily complete absence of any threat to the self-structure' (Rogers, 1951, p.517). If this can be sustained, it will lead to the person 'self-righting' and the fault lines will be sealed with new, trustworthy self-accredited experiences. If a superficial quick fix is applied, the fault lines remain, ready to be activated by new challenging life experiences.

What is so different about this approach is that person-centred theory says there is a single type of cause for all distress. This single cause, though, finds an unlimited number of ways of expressing itself, because each person, and their experience, is different. This makes any one person's trajectory of distress completely unpredictable unless their effort is turned 100% to finding the meaning of the experiences with the best expert available – the person themself. Such a theory is completely antagonistic to any kind of system of categories or diagnosis, including the medical model. It also means that person-centred literature is not crowded with books and articles on how to treat this problem or that diagnosis differentially. For professionals who think that complicated diagnostic categories and expert-driven treatment protocols are a sign of sophistication, this leaves the person-centred approach looking lightweight and naïve.

Before Rogers, professional therapy relationships were cast in the mould of the powerful expert doctor and helpless patient lacking insight. Rogers' work made it possible for lay people (non-medically qualified) and other professionals to work much more as companions in a person-to-person way – something that many of us now see as essential (but, sadly, still cannot be taken for granted). Rogers was not only a pioneer of the importance of the relationship in therapy; he was the first to record a complete therapy relationship onto wax discs, publish a word-for-word transcript and initiate research into the effectiveness of psychotherapy, including looking at individual interventions (for more about Carl Rogers, see Kirschenbaum, 2007; for more about research, see Cooper et al., 2010).

Conclusion

We hope this brief trip through some of the main psychological theories has helped you to figure out some new ways to think about your problems, or those of a loved one. Or maybe one or two of them just confirm what you already thought. We suggest you don't try too hard to figure out which is the best theory. There is a lot of overlap between them. For example, are the defence mechanisms that Freud talks about really so different from the 'faulty thinking' described by the cognitive theorists? They are both examples of how we distort or misperceive ourselves and the world around us.

Perhaps all the theories have something to offer at different times in your life. If there is a common message, it is perhaps that we aren't born with the problems we have as adults; they aren't somehow inherently and inevitably built into our brains. Rather, they come from our interactions with other people, especially, but not exclusively, early on in life.

We now move on to look at how the causes identified in Chapter 6 and the theories discussed in this chapter apply to the most common problem of all, experienced by most of us at some time in our lives – depression.

Chapter 8
Putting things together: formulating depression

Formulation is a process that an increasing number of mental health professionals use to put together and make sense of the information they gather during formal assessment, and from other sources, in order to create a systematic, positive framework of understanding and action to help the client. A crucial element of formulation is positively acting on the fact that, for many clients, their own understanding of the difficulties that they or their relatives experience can be the key to making positive changes in their lives.

For many professionals, formulation is replacing diagnosis as the main framework for making sense of their clients' experiences. One of the aims is to empower people by identifying, in partnership with them, a shared understanding of the origins of their difficulties and negotiating areas for change and development. This is in contrast to simple diagnosis and prescription of treatment, which often leaves people feeling dependent on professionals to solve their difficulties. We will describe a very new and increasingly influential development in the field of formulation, the Power Threat Meaning Framework, in Chapter 9.

Developing understanding by using formulation as a method

In order to show how the causes listed in Chapter 6 and the psychological theories described in Chapter 7 can work together to understand a 'mental health problem', an example may be helpful. We thought it would be a good idea to continue with our example of depression. It is the most common diagnosis. One in six people in the UK will suffer from an experience that would be classified as depression at some point in their life. The number of new diagnosed cases of depression worldwide increased from 172 million in 1990 to 258 million in 2017 – an increase of 50% (Liu et al., 2020).

In addition, many people whose primary problem is something else (anxiety, eating disorders, drug and alcohol problems, psychosis and so on) are also likely to have what would be regarded as symptoms of depression.

Diagnosis is not a formulation

Many psychiatrists argue that there is a difference between ordinary depression, or sadness, and what they call 'major depression', which they consider to be a disorder or a mental illness. The *DSM* (see Chapter 4) has a way of separating those who just feel depressed from those who have this thing called 'major depressive disorder' (MDD). It does so by what some have called the 'smorgasbord approach to diagnosis'. This involves listing some behaviours and feelings and then saying you need a certain number of them to be categorised as having the thing in question. To be labelled as having MDD, you need any five of the following nine 'symptoms':

- depressed mood
- loss of interest in things that normally give you pleasure
- weight loss or gain
- sleeping difficulties
- agitation or slowing down of movement responses
- fatigue or loss of energy
- feelings of worthlessness or guilt
- concentration or decision-making difficulties
- suicidal thoughts.

For this particular diagnosis, you need to have had these five (or more) symptoms for most of the time almost every day for at least two weeks.

A diagnosis from an appropriately qualified mental health professional can be useful for managers of mental health services who have to decide how to allocate limited resources. In some countries, a diagnosis is essential if the person is to access services or funding for services. People with a diagnosis like MDD are, therefore, likely to get help; those who do not meet the criteria (who have, say, only four out of nine 'symptoms') may be less likely to get help. But this process is useless when it comes to deciding whether a person is 'actually depressed' or not. The real world of human emotions does not fit into neat little boxes and, as we hope we have shown in previous chapters, emotions are incredibly difficult to define, in terms of generalised experience.

Depression (and anxiety, and most other problems) is not a category of experience that anyone can say with confidence that some of us have and some of us do not. At best, it is a dimension or continuum of experience along which we all vary from month to month, day to day, and sometimes even hour to hour. Naturally, we would expect some folk to have a broader range of movement up and down this dimension. Others spend too much time at the more depressed end of the dimension. But to claim that some of us have something called 'depression' and some of us don't is an argument that's difficult to sustain.

If we believe we have something called 'depression' or 'MDD', then it's all too easy to start also believing that this thing, this disorder or mental illness, is actually somehow causing us to feel depressed. People who think like this are likely to answer the question, 'Why are you feeling depressed?' with, 'Because I have MDD'. Regardless of the absence of logic, we are invited to believe that the symptoms in the list used to decide who has this thing called MDD are supposedly caused by the label given to people who have five or more of them. For example, 'Different people are affected in different ways by major depression. Some people have trouble sleeping, they lose weight, and they generally feel agitated and irritable.' This is a circular argument that actually explains nothing about the causes of the experiences that we might label as feeling depressed. It does create a situation where everyone concerned (from the person in question through to the mental health professionals working with them) need not bother to try to figure out what has really caused them to feel so down and what changes might be needed (in thinking, feeling, behaviour or living conditions) in order to feel better. Some people are happy with this sort of approach to understanding the causes of 'depression', since the reassurance (we repeat, regardless of the absence of logic) can be comforting.

Sources of information for formulations

Biological factors

We have seen how, in recent years, depression, like everything else, has received much attention from genetic researchers. There is evidence that depression runs in families (Klein et al., 2001). There is also evidence that, when people are depressed, the neurotransmitters in their brain (especially serotonin and norepinephrine) are either at a low level or are out of balance with each other (Rampello et al., 2000), and metabolism is slower in certain parts of the brain (Schatzberg, 2002).

However, we have already argued that, just because problems, including depression, run in families does not mean there is a genetic component (Joseph, 2022a). It can be depressing growing up with depressed parents – either because Mom and Dad are too preoccupied or sad to give us what we need as kids and/or because we learn to copy their way of dealing with problems. We have also argued, however, that everything is an interaction between our genes and our environment. We just don't believe there is any good evidence that there is a specific genetic predisposition to specific mental health problems. Probably the most important thing we inherit genetically is a greater or lesser sensitivity to stress in general. But even so, it is hard to say, at birth for instance, what is genetic and what is the result of Mom being stressed during pregnancy. We have argued too that there isn't a whole lot we can do about our genetic make-up and that it is more useful, therefore, to focus on the depressing things (and our reactions to them) that have caused our depression and figure out which ones we can do something about.

It has also been proposed that, when people are depressed, the neurotransmitters in their brain (especially serotonin) may be at a low level. We have already noted, however, that a recent analysis of 17 previous reviews of serotonin-depression research found 'no consistent evidence of there being an association between serotonin and depression, and no support for the hypothesis that depression is caused by lowered serotonin activity or concentrations' (Moncrieff et al., 2022).

We have also already argued that, just because our brains function differently when we are depressed, it does not mean there is something wrong with our brains that has somehow caused 'the depression'. Our brains are simply responding to depressing events.

So the kinds of biological factors focused on by the 'medical model' are not usually helpful when developing a formulation. Of course, more substantive biologically based issues, like physical illness, disabilities, head injury and so on, in oneself or in loved ones, may well be important to include.

External causes

In Chapter 6 we looked at some of the research studies proving that the public is right (Chapter 5) to assume that depression (like other mental health problems) is primarily caused by depressing things happening in our lives. For example, you may remember the study covering 14 USA states that found that admission to hospital for depression was significantly predicted by poverty and unemployment (Fortney et al., 2007). Other environmental or external events that can help cause depression include childhood abuse (emotional, physical and sexual) and child neglect, bullying in school, violence, including rape, being an immigrant or member of an ethic minority (especially if you are poor and/or experience discrimination) and loss.

Loss, of course, is a strong candidate as a cause of depression. We have seen (in Chapter 6) that loss comes in many shapes and sizes and is an inevitable part of being human. We have discussed why, when they experience, for instance, the loss of a cherished partner or a job they valued, some people seem to cope with the sadness and others seem to get stuck in a very deep feeling of hopelessness about the future. Some of the things that make the difference are other external factors, including previous losses, level of support from friends and family and our general quality of life beyond who or what we have just lost. We have also seen, however, that internal factors, including what we tell ourselves about the loss, are also hugely important.

Internal causes

Believing (for whatever reason) that your feelings are caused by an imagined irreversible chemical imbalance in your brain, or faulty genes, or a 'mental illness' called 'Major Depressive Disorder', while possibly reassuring that it's 'not your fault', is not particularly motivating. Empowering individual people in their struggle with distress and disturbing experiences is a tricky thing – balancing reassurance and hope with challenging 'home truths'. We have explained that we understand why so many people find diagnosis reassuring, or even a lifeline in desperate times, but we are convinced that simply diagnosing experiences using arbitrary labels is unhelpful in the long run.

Some beliefs are born out of our efforts to cope with our experiences – some of these will be helpful and some will not. In truth, it's very difficult for anyone on the 'outside' of the experiences to know what will be helpful to any particular client. The skill is to work in a consultative partnership with the client to find out what helps, what hinders, what is harmful and what is positive. In our summary of cognitive theory in Chapter 7, we looked at a range of other unhelpful things we tell ourselves that can cause or exacerbate feeling depressed.

For many mental health professions, cognitive theory has become a very popular way to understand and treat depression (see Chapter 7). Blaming ourselves when depressing things happen is all too easy to do – especially when we are little. At certain stages in their emotional and cognitive development, children tend to think everything is to do with them. So as a child, when anything bad (or good for that matter) happens, we think we must be responsible. If Mom and Dad split up, a five-year-old can easily assume that it is something they did, or didn't do, that caused it, unless Mom and Dad go out of their way to explain otherwise and demonstrate it in their behaviour. Even when we are grown up, we can still sometimes feel overly responsible for things.

Although cognitive theory can be helpful in understanding and overcoming depression, other theories can also help our understanding. In terms of psychodynamic and humanistic theories, we might ask whether our parents were so focused on teaching us right from wrong that they forgot to make sure we felt loved for ourselves, regardless of our behaviour. Did they give us the impression that they only loved us if we achieved well at school, or fulfilled their aspirations for us? Attachment theory would have us consider if events in early life meant that we couldn't establish that essential safe and trusting primary relationship in our first few years.

Did we learn early on in life, from our main role models, to withdraw from others and close down emotionally whenever something depressing happens, as might be suggested by social learning theory? Or did we simply learn to stop doing the things that make us feel good when we first start feeling a bit down, producing a downward spiral?

Positives as well as negatives

There is a tendency among mental health professionals to focus on the negative. First, we list all the 'pathological' behaviours or thoughts that someone has and then, having applied the appropriate label, we go in search of bad things to explain the bad behaviours – whether they be dysfunctional brains, faulty genes, unhappy childhoods or whatever. Life is not really like that. Life is, of course, a combination of good and bad. So, when trying to understand another human being (or ourselves), we need to factor in the positives. From a practical point of view, in terms of what helps when we are depressed, it can be very important to focus on our existing strengths, so they can be valued and nurtured, as well as on the things (external and internal) that we might want to change. A famous psychologist, George Albee (1921–2006), came up with a rather simple equation for thinking about the chances of developing depression or other mental health problems (Albee, 1985):

$$\text{Chances of mental health problem} = \frac{\text{Organic factors} + \text{stress} + \text{exploitation}}{\text{Coping skills} + \text{self-esteem} + \text{support groups}}$$

Other authors, writing about how to prevent psychosis, have explained:

To reduce the incidence of madness, we must increase the size of the denominator [below the line] and decrease the size of the numerator [above the line]. This requires reducing our exposure to stressful or traumatic events and increasing our capacity to participate fully in the world by creating a more just society. At the same time, it involves increasing our ability to cope with trauma and inequity, by learning better coping skills, enhancing our self-esteem and developing better formal and informal social support systems. (Davies & Burdett, 2004)

Putting it all together – the formulation

In training programmes across a range of disciplines around the world, students are taught to 'formulate' – to attempt to put all the information about a person's mental health problem together. So far in this chapter, we have tried to put some flesh on the bones of the idea that the type of formulation you come up with depends on what sort of information you have got to work with and what sort of model you have in mind. As we suggested at the start of the chapter, if you are working from a 'medical model' and only know what 'symptoms' a person has, you come up with nothing more than a 'diagnostic formulation', which is really just a fancy term for a label. If, however, you have taken a thorough psychosocial history (covering the sorts of things discussed in Chapter 6), and you have some understanding of psychological theories (Chapter 7), you come up with something much more interesting and, potentially, much more useful.

A psychological formulation tries to explain a problem like depression in terms of the person's life history. It tries, however, to go beyond just listing all the depressing things that have happened. The goal is to answer the question, '*How* did those things lead to someone feeling hopeless about the future'? It is also, therefore, addressing the question why, after the death of their husband (say), this person, the client or patient in front of us, ended up severely depressed when others who suffer a similar loss do not.

There are many ways to approach a formulation. One way is to break things down into predisposing factors, precipitating factors, perpetuating factors and preventative factors (the 'four Ps'). Predisposing factors tend to be things that happened earlier in life that increase the chances of getting very depressed when, later in life, a depressing thing happens (the precipitating factor). Predisposing factors can be external events – such as child abuse or early loss of a parent, but they include internal processes – such as learning early on in life to blame yourself for everything that goes wrong, to dislike yourself, to be scared of close relationships and so on. A precipitating factor is anything that pushes you over the edge, sometimes by triggering one or more of your predisposing factors. So, someone with a lot of early losses – or one huge early loss – can sometimes become very depressed when faced with another loss later in life.

Perpetuating factors are, as the term implies, anything that tends to maintain the problem, such as chronic stressors, poverty, unsupportive family and so on, or internal factors, such as telling yourself you are unlovable. Preventative factors are the strengths that a person has despite all their problems, internal (skills and so on) and external (such as support from friends and family and a good job).

Formulations are usually done at the level of the individual person, although it can be invaluable (although more complicated) to formulate a group – a family, for instance.) If you, or a loved one, are sometimes (or often) depressed, it might be helpful to try to list the predisposing, precipitating, perpetuating and preventive factors involved. Table 8.1 lists some examples of the four Ps in relation to depression.

Then, using one or more of the models (pick the ones that make most sense to you – or make up your own model), try to fit it all together. Figure 8.1 illustrates one possibility. There is no totally complete or correct formulation, so don't worry about getting it 'right'. It's a way of having a constructive dialogue with yourself about your experiences. Some of the connections you make in undertaking this exercise may jump out at you as making sense.

Of course, many readers will have already been doing this for years. We all have our formulations of our problems (and other people's). We just don't call them formulations. Any case study submitted in training by a student that has a thorough and sensible formulation but does not include the client's own formulation should be returned to them as incomplete.

Table 8.1: Some examples of the four Ps in relation to depression

Predisposing (in past)	Precipitating (recent)	Perpetuating (current/ongoing)	Preventative (current/ongoing)
External	*External*	*External*	*External*
Childhood neglect	Loss (person, job etc.)	No friends	Supportive family
Childhood abuse	Failure	Critical family/friends	Supportive friends
Bullying	Physical abuse	Work stress	Satisfying job
Depressed parent(s)	Emotional abuse	Unemployment	Children
Deaths in family	Financial problems	Poverty	
Other losses	Other depressing events	Parenting stress	
		Violence	
Poverty			
Discrimination			
Internal	*Internal*	*Internal*	*Internal*
Blaming self for any of the above	Realisation dreams or goals not being attained	Hopeless about future	Hope for the future
Learning to distrust other people	Humiliating failure at work	Dislike of self	A plan
Feeling loved only if we live up to others' expectations	Failure of relationship	Fear of other people	Liking self

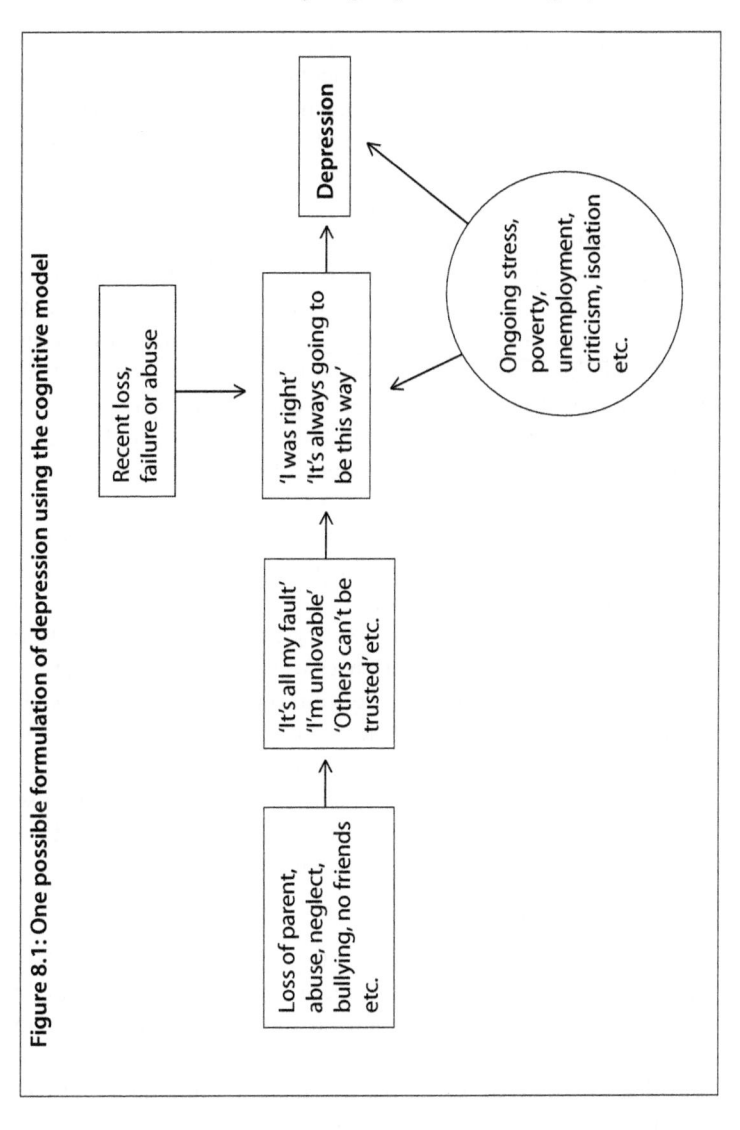

Figure 8.1: One possible formulation of depression using the cognitive model

Loss of parent, abuse, neglect, bullying, no friends etc. → 'It's all my fault' 'I'm unlovable' 'Others can't be trusted' etc. → 'I was right' 'It's always going to be this way' → **Depression**

Recent loss, failure or abuse → 'I was right' 'It's always going to be this way'

Ongoing stress, poverty, unemployment, criticism, isolation etc.

Mental health professionals often forget that clients already have their own theories about what is causing, and maintaining, the problem. Sometimes, however, the client's formulation has been part of the problem – a perpetuating factor in its own right. If a client's formulation of why they feel depressed so much of the time is that they are somehow a bad person who deserves to feel so wretched, or that they have a mental illness called 'depressive disorder' about which nothing much can be done – then that needs some further thought. Some formulations are less helpful than others.

So, while it simply can't be the case in mental health services that the 'customer is always right', it is absolutely essential that all practitioners (from support workers to consultant psychologists and psychiatrists) listen respectfully to the client's formulation. Being respectful includes sharing one's own formulation with the client and then talking about any differences between the two. There are almost always differences. Two heads are invariably better than one when trying to understand something as complicated as a human being – especially when one of the heads is the subject of the formulation.

So, in trying to understand the causes of a person's 'depression', we think good practice requires the professional to ask the patient or client what their formulation is, and if they don't have one, to try to construct one. If you are reading this book and wondering about whether your own experiences would add up to a diagnosis of 'depression', why not try making your own formulation instead? Then check it out with a couple of people who know you well: what do they think? Make sure you choose these people well. They need to be people whose judgement you trust but who are also able to be honest with you. Don't take their views as 'the truth' – theirs are just additional perspectives to be considered.

A word of caution

If you are reading this book in order to gain a better understanding of your own experiences or of someone close to you, you should proceed with caution. A quick look at Table 8.1 should be enough to make us realise that we all have a range of precipitating factors, and that for some of us the list will include thinking about bad experiences in the past. How sensitive we are to memories as precipitating factors will depend on the sort of person we are. We all react in different ways. For some, formulation will be a positive, empowering discovery; for others it might be a trigger for a mildly disturbing but handleable experience. For a few it might be akin to reliving a trauma or abuse.

If you can guess beforehand that trying your own formulation will trigger distress or re-traumatise you, either don't do it or attempt it only with support from a trusted friend or professional. The next chapter will summarise our arguments and highlight several encouraging developments.

Chapter 9
2010–2022 and looking to the future: a call for action

As we have argued in this book, we need a very different, non-medical understanding of distress, one that sees it as arising out of people's lives and the sense they make of what has happened to them. Chapter 6 described how traumas and adversities are likely to lead to mental health problems of all kinds. Chapter 8 showed how we can put this information together and create personal stories, or 'formulations', which can serve as an alternative to diagnosis.

We want to end here with a summary of some very important international (global) developments that we believe are game-changers and route markers in the move towards a better, humane way of understanding the 'causes of mental health problems'.

Trauma-informed approaches

The first is the gradual but growing adoption of 'trauma-informed' approaches (TIAs) in mental health services, which is happening on a worldwide scale. We prefer a broad definition of 'trauma', one that includes ongoing adversities as well as one-off events. TIAs are:

> informed by neuroscience, psychology and social science as well as attachment and trauma theories, and give central prominence to the complex and pervasive impact trauma has on a person's worldview and interrelationships. (Sweeney et al., 2016)

In other words, this is an approach that understands the causes of mental health problems to be multifactorial and demands that treatments address that fact (including recognising the potentially traumatising effects of traditional psychiatric interventions and environments, on staff as well as patients).

To this end, as Sweeney and colleagues state in their comprehensive discussion paper (2016):

> First and foremost, a paradigm shift in collective thinking about the causes of mental distress is vital. Practitioners must move from asking 'what is wrong with you' to 'what happened to you'. In other words, practitioners must understand the critical and primary role of trauma and fundamentally change their practice as a result.

Alongside, they state, there needs to be 'system-wide change' and, most importantly:

> We believe that trauma survivors have a pivotal role to play in this. We live the impact of trauma every day. We understand its devastating effects, the damage inflicted by the current mental health system, the need for mutual relationships based on safety and cooperation, the need for personal control, and the vital support of peers. (Sweeney et al., 2016)

The Power Threat Meaning Framework

The second is a new way of conceptualising why people sometimes experience a whole range of forms of distress, confusion, fear, despair and troubled or troubling behaviour. The Power Threat Meaning Framework (Johnstone & Boyle et al., 2018) builds on formulation and trauma-informed practice, and draws heavily on the evidence summarised in this book so far.

It is by far the biggest breakthrough for years in terms of understanding causal factors, and is the result of several years' work by a group of British mental health professionals and 'service users', led by prominent clinical psychologists Professor Mary Boyle and Dr Lucy Johnstone. We are very grateful that Lucy agreed to outline for us here the Power Threat Meaning Framework:

The Power Threat Meaning Framework (PTMF), published in 2018 by the British Psychological Society, is an alternative to the more traditional models based on psychiatric diagnosis (Johnstone et al., 2018). It was co-produced with service users and applies not just to people who have been in contact with the mental health or criminal justice systems but to all of us. This is because all of us face difficulties in our lives at some point, all of us struggle at times, and all of us have to find ways of managing the resulting distress. Thus, the PTMF does not believe there is a separate group of people who are 'mentally ill', or have 'mental health problems'.

A popular survivor slogan is 'Instead of asking what's wrong with me, ask what's happened to me.' The PTMF takes this question as its starting point, and expands it with a set of additional questions, which can apply to individuals, families or social groups:

- 'What has happened to you?' (How is **Power** operating in your life?)
- 'How did it affect you?' (What kind of **Threats** does this pose?)
- 'What sense did you make of it?' (What is the **Meaning** of these situations and experiences to you?)
- 'What did you have to do to survive?' (What kinds of **Threat Response** are you using?)

In addition, the two questions below help us to think about what skills and resources people might have and how we might pull all these ideas and responses together into a personal narrative or story:

- 'What are your strengths?' (What access to **Power resources** do you have?)
- 'What is your story?' (How does all this fit together?)

The questions do not have to be asked in those words or in that order. They are simply an overlapping set of prompts to start us thinking about the various aspects of people's difficulties. They can be used as a rough structure for creating more hopeful narratives or stories about people's lives and the difficulties they may have faced or are still facing, instead of seeing themselves as blameworthy, weak, deficient or 'mentally ill'.

In order to help people think about these questions, the PTMF summarises a great deal of evidence about the role of various kinds of power in people's lives; the kinds of threat that misuses of power pose to us, and the ways we have learned as human beings to respond to threat. In trauma-informed practice, these responses are often referred to as 'survival strategies' – necessary at the time, but which can outlive their usefulness and gradually become problematic of themselves. For example, people sometimes dissociate or cut off from traumatic events, but the suppressed feelings may later emerge in the form of hostile voices. In traditional mental health practice, these threat responses are called 'symptoms'.

In addition, the PTMF places a great deal of emphasis on a form of power we are less used to thinking about – ideological power. This refers to the ability of some groups in society, often those who already enjoy greater advantages, to support certain interests through the language we are encouraged to use, the assumptions we make and the meanings we create. For example, politicians may use terms like 'welfare scroungers' about the unemployed, in contrast to 'wealth-creators' – and in doing so, they may make it easier to impose harsh conditions on the jobless and justify the privileges of those who already enjoy a great deal of material and economic power.

Ideological power is often expressed through social expectations and standards, which are reinforced through education, the media and in many other ways. If we believe certain definitions of success, which in Western societies are often based on competition and material possessions, then we are likely to feel a sense of failure if we are unable to live up to them. Similarly, if we are encouraged to stereotype and discriminate against particular ethnic or cultural groups, those people will face barriers to participating fully in society and may even begin to see themselves as less deserving. By examining the influence of ideological power, the PTMF helps us to understand how all of us, even if we have not experienced specific traumas or abuses, can end up feeling full of shame, self-blame, isolation, fear and guilt.

From a PTMF perspective, imposing a psychiatric label on someone can be seen as an example of the operation of ideological power. As we have discussed, these labels are not scientifically valid, and yet they often shape people's lives in very damaging ways. People are not usually offered alternatives, and if they protest or disagree, they may find themselves subjected to other kinds of power, such as forced psychiatric drugs. However, the diagnostic model of distress arguably serves the interests of professionals, drug companies and, to an extent, society as a whole, as we are all shielded from looking too closely at the real root causes of distress.

A peer group that used the PTMF questions as a way to support each other to construct their own narratives reported that:

> We found that the Framework is applicable to many forms of adversity, even where there is no history of overt trauma, such as sudden unemployment or homelessness, stigma and discrimination, or even adapting to life-changing circumstances such as health difficulties etc... Members were able to use the supportive peer-led environment to develop their narratives without professional support. Through sharing and reflecting on their experiences, they developed insight into how disempowerment, threats to autonomy and many other misuses of power had impacted negatively on their lives and often continued to play out in the present. They welcomed the description of their reactions as normal human responses to challenging and traumatic events and circumstances... We found that sharing experiences... is an emotive and thought-provoking way to connect with others... and this may be the first time that the narrative and pain have truly been heard... This takes us from being isolated and lonely individuals to being part of a wider community of equals. (Griffiths, 2019)

The PTMF uses the term 'narrative' to include not just formulation but any kind of meaning-making, whether inside or outside services, including art, music, poetry, community myths, rituals and ceremonies. It is well known that experiences and expressions of distress are often very different around the globe and in minority groups in the UK. The *DSM* response to this puzzling (from a medical viewpoint) fact is to try to translate these forms of distress back into the diagnostic model. The PTMF, on the other hand, encourages respect for non-Western, non-medical ways of expressing and healing distress, which are often narrative-based, and which may be very effective in their own cultural context.

The PTMF is an over-arching framework that is not intended to replace all the ways we currently think about and work with distress. Instead, the aim is to support and strengthen the many examples of good practice that already exist, while also suggesting new ways forward. These may or may not involve therapy and other standard interventions, including, if they help someone to cope, psychiatric drugs. For others, their main needs will be for practical help and resources, perhaps along with peer support, art, music, exercise, nutrition, community activism and so on. More widely, the PTMF suggests alternatives in all the various forums where diagnosis is currently used, such as service design and commissioning, professional training, research, service user involvement and public information.

One of the main purposes of the PTMF is to highlight the links between individual distress and socio-economic policies, and the way that social inequalities and injustices play out in our lives. In this way, it has implications well beyond services. It shows that distress cannot be healed purely at a personal level while our social contexts and values remain so damaging and our society is so fragmented and unequal. The PTMF perspective on distress takes us beyond the individual and shows that we are all part of a wider struggle for a fairer society.

The PTMF authors have been encouraged by the very enthusiastic response to the document. In the UK there are pilot studies in some services and charities, and it is taught on some training courses. It has also been taken up in peer groups. There has been interest from a number of other countries, and six translations are now in progress. All this will feed back into further development of the Framework.[1]

---

1. You can access the PTMF documents, along with videos, podcasts, good practice examples, training materials and other resources at www.bps.org.uk/member-networks/division-clinical-psychology/power-threat-meaning-framework

A set of prompts for constructing your own PTMF narrative can be found under 'suggested guided discussion document' on the main PTMF webpage: www.bps.org.uk/member-networks/division-clinical-psychology/power-threat-meaning-framework

A fuller but summarised description of the PTMF can be found in a recent addition to this Straight Talking series, *The Straight Talking Introduction to the Power Threat Meaning Framework* (Boyle & Johnstone, 2020).

Covid-19 and its aftermath

The third major development is one of the very few positives that have emerged from the massive, far-reaching and deeply challenging events of the past 10 years.

The world is a very different place to what it was when the first edition of our book appeared in 2010. So many unpredictable and/or shocking events have taken place, including the election of Donald Trump as President of the USA and Boris Johnson, followed by Liz Truss, as Prime Minister in the UK; the UK leaving the European Union; the rise of the far right across Europe; the rapidly worsening climate crisis; wars in Syria, Yemen and, most recently, the Russian invasion of Ukraine, and more than 6.5 million people killed worldwide by the Covid-19 pandemic. If, like us, you believe that bad things happen and make us unhappy, all of these, and their economic, social and political consequences, will of course have majorly impacted on people's mental health. We think it is interesting to explore this here, in terms of furthering our understanding of the causes of mental health problems.

Let's take as an example the effects of Covid-19 on our mental health. In early 2020, while the UK population was stocking up on pasta and toilet paper, a team of researchers was setting in place an 18-month project to monitor the psychological, social, economic and political impact of the pandemic on the general population.

The COVID-19 Psychological Research Consortium Study, led by Professor Richard Bentall, co-editor of this *Straight Talking Introduction* series, recruited a representative sample of more than 2,000 UK adults and collected information, at intervals, on:

> their psychological and physical health, their engagement with social distancing and other hygienic practices, their thoughts and beliefs in relation to a potential vaccine for COVID-19, their political views, as well as their level of satisfaction in relation to how their government is managing the crisis. (McBride et al., 2021)

This remarkable project has led to more than 60 publications so far, all freely available to the public.[2] We will look at just two of

---

2. www.sheffield.ac.uk/psychology-consortium-covid19/publications

them here. The first, entitled 'Anxiety, depression, traumatic stress and COVID-19-related anxiety in the UK general population during the COVID-19 pandemic,' was conducted over the week beginning 23 March 2020, 52 days after the first confirmed Covid-19 case in the UK and the day Boris Johnson, then Prime Minister, announced the first 'lockdown' that required all people in the UK not to leave their homes except for very limited purposes (Shevlin et al., 2020).

The survey found higher levels of anxiety and depression compared with pre-Covid population studies, 'but not dramatically so'. Anxiety or depression were specifically predicted by younger age, living with children, high estimates of personal risk, low income, loss of income and pre-existing health conditions in self and others. The researchers concluded:

> The fact that the prevalence of psychological problems observed in the present study was not dramatically higher than those reported in previous studies suggests that the population, at an early stage of the pandemic, has successfully adapted to the unprecedented changes that have been forced on their lifestyles. However, we have identified certain key groups who may be more vulnerable to the social and economic challenges of the pandemic, particularly those whose income has been affected, who have children living in the home and who have pre-existing health conditions that make them vulnerable to the more devastating effects of the COVID-19 virus. (Shevlin et al., 2020)

These minimal increases in anxiety and depression among certain social groups only stood in stark contrast to ominous warnings of a 'tsunami' of referrals for mental illness from the Royal College of Psychiatrists in May 2020.[3] Indeed, the second paper we will discuss here from the COVID-19 Psychological Research Consortium Study was entitled 'Refuting the myth of a 'tsunami' of mental ill-health in populations affected by COVID-19: Evidence that response to the pandemic is heterogeneous, not homogeneous.' It reported data at three time points (Shevlin et al., 2021).

---

3. www.bbc.co.uk/news/health-52676981

This reported that, overall prevalence of anxiety-depression had remained stable, while Covid-related trauma symptoms had reduced over time, perhaps because of 'habituation to the situation'. It identified three groups, categorised as reflecting stability, deterioration and improvement. The majority of the sample 'exhibited resilient mental health trajectories... characterised by minimal changes in anxious-depressive or PTSD symptomology'. This suggested that, although some individuals may exhibit long-term distress following traumatic/adverse events, resilience (maintaining healthy outcomes or 'bouncing back' following such events) is the most common and consistently observed response. About 5% of the sample studied reported severe psychological distress during the first months of lockdown, and about 8% reported improvement in psychological wellbeing.

This time the researchers concluded:

> The emergence of both improving and deteriorating classes in the current study suggests that, while it may have taken several months for some individuals to adjust and adapt to the situation, for others, deterioration may have only emerged after months of increased caring duties, balancing home and work life, or with the end of the furlough scheme looming. (Shevlin et al., 2021)

One of us (John) wrote in his regular blog for *Psychology Today*:

> Some might characterise the outcomes been measured by Bentall and his colleagues as 'mental illnesses' or 'psychiatric disorders' supposedly caused by biochemical imbalances and genetic predispositions, and supposedly requiring psychiatric drugs. What this impressive body of work shows, however, is that our reactions to the pandemic are exactly that – understandable, emotional reactions to distressing life events. The image I am left with is not of a tsunami of people with mental illnesses but of a young couple (or single parent) with three young kids at home who have just lost, or are about to lose, their meagre income. Of course they are scared. Of course they have days when all seems hopeless. Targeting the causes of their fear and hopelessness will help them more

than applying a scientifically dubious diagnostic label to their emotions (Anxiety Disorder, Major Depressive Episode etc.) and recommending a medical solution. (Read, 2021)

Thus, we have a mass of evidence showing that, when bad things happen, they can indeed make us unhappy, but that we do, in most cases, have the ability to adapt and respond using our ordinary, everyday resources, if we are fortunate enough to have them. It's what we've done throughout the story of humankind – how else would humans have survived?

Seismic shifts in international policy

And last, two very important international bodies have now proclaimed very clear positions on the causes of mental health problems. In 2019, the United Nations Human Rights Council (UNHRC) published a report by its 'special rapporteur on the right to health', Lithuanian psychiatrist Dr Dainius Pūras. He stated categorically the link between mental health problems and external environmental influences, and deplored the 'medicalisation' of 'normal reactions to life's many pressures'. He wrote:

> Current mental health policies have been affected to a large extent by the asymmetry of power and biases because of the dominance of the biomedical model and biomedical interventions. This model has led not only to the overuse of coercion in case of psychosocial, intellectual and cognitive disabilities, but also to the medicalization of normal reactions to life's many pressures, including moderate forms of social anxiety, sadness, shyness, truancy and antisocial behaviour... This message may further the excessive use of diagnostic categories and expand the medical model to diagnose pathologies and provide individual treatment modalities that lead to excessive medicalization. The message diverts policies and practices from embracing two powerful modern approaches: a public health approach and a human rights-based approach.... Overmedicalization is especially harmful to children, and global trends to medicalize complex psychosocial and public health issues in childhood should be addressed with a stronger political will. (UNHRC, 2019)

Two years later the World Health Organization published a 300-page document entitled *Guidance on Community Mental Health Services: Promoting person-centred and rights-based approaches* (WHO, 2021). It argued:

> The predominant focus of care in many contexts continues to be on diagnosis, medication and symptom reduction. Critical social determinants that impact on people's mental health such as violence, discrimination, poverty, exclusion, isolation, job insecurity or unemployment, lack of access to housing, social safety nets, and health services, are often overlooked or excluded from mental health concepts and practice. This leads to an over-diagnosis of human distress and over-reliance on psychotropic drugs to the detriment of psychosocial interventions.

The report cited 22 recent international examples where mental health services were working differently, developing psychosocial interventions that recognised the primacy of the person's experience in understanding their problems. They include the Finnish model of Open Dialogue, now being adopted in many other countries,[4] the Soteria approach,[5] and Hearing Voices peer-support groups.[6]

A psychiatrist changes his mind

These ideas are also increasingly finding backing from within mainstream psychiatry. Sir Robin Murray is the UK's leading psychiatric schizophrenia researcher, and was, for a long time, a committed adherent to the medical model of mental 'illness'. In 2017, he bravely wrote an article titled 'Mistakes I Have Made in My Research Career', in which he declared:

> Asthma may be a lung disease but it is one which can be precipitated by environmental toxins (eg. pollution) and allergens. Just as the lungs process air, so the brain processes

---

4. https://open-dialogue.net

5. www.soterianetwork.org.uk

6. www.hearing-voices.org

external stimuli; consequently, its healthy function can be harmed by noxious factors in the social environment such as childhood abuse or adverse life events... In the last two decades, it has become obvious that child abuse, urbanization, migration, and adverse life events contribute to the etiology of schizophrenia and other psychoses. This has been a big shift for me!... My preconceptions had made me blind to the influence of the social environment. (Murray, 2017)

Murray also invited John to write an editorial for *Psychological Medicine*, the respected psychiatric journal he edits, critiquing psychiatry's 'medical model' of depression. John and psychiatrist Joanna Moncrieff wrote in 'Depression: Why drugs and electricity are not the answer' (Read & Moncrieff, 2022):

Viewing depression as a medical disorder that somehow originates in the brain and responds to brain-based interventions is fundamentally inconsistent with understanding it as a 'normal' human emotion, albeit sometimes extreme and disproportionate – that is as a meaningful reaction to depressing circumstances. Although we will focus on the failure to establish that antidepressants and ECT are effective or safe, we do so from the perspective that this approach, focussed as it is on decontextualized, pathologised, individuals or brains, is flawed from the outset. For example, it cannot address the issues underlying women being about twice as likely as men to receive either 'treatment'. We are not alone in calling instead for approaches that acknowledge the meaning of depression, and address the common social origins of misery and sadness.

Final words

Hopefully, this book has offered some useful ways to think about what might have led to some of the difficult thoughts, emotions or behaviours in your life, or in the lives of those you love. It is also to be hoped that new understandings will lead to new approaches to those problems. At the very least, these new understandings about causes may make your difficulties less bewildering and reduce the chances that you blame yourself, or something unalterable inside you, for them.

We have seen that there are lots of possible reasons why some of us sometimes feel extremely overwhelmed, frightened, distressed, depressed or confused. There are also lots of different theories about how this long list of precipitating factors can impact on us, and within us, to bring about these problems. Perhaps that is the most important lesson from all this: that there is no single right answer to the question, 'What causes mental health problems?' And the lesson resulting from that is that we should be wary of anyone, expert or friend, who tells us they know what is the cause of our problem, and especially if they tell us that it is one thing alone (biological, social or psychological).

Genes, brain chemicals, childhood abuse, even the most painful early loss are not by themselves likely to be the whole answer. It is usually a combination of factors, past and present, external and internal. It is complicated, but not so complicated that it isn't worth trying to figure out the major factors and how they may be interacting. You stand a good chance of finding out some of the causes, and in almost all cases will learn something potentially useful. However, this involves not only a bit of thinking but also, often, some feeling too. Digging around in the past can be messy.

Perhaps that is why diagnoses and simplistic biological theories are so attractive. They are not only simple, they can also be relatively pain free. So, when thinking about the causes of mental health problems, people may have to be prepared to do some feeling too. Sometimes the thoughts and feelings they discover will turn out not to be 'mental health problems' at all, just understandable emotional reactions to things that have happened. It might also be the case that they need to do a little more work on accepting certain feelings as normal and a little less work on changing – which may come from labelling something a 'problem'. So, paradoxically, and in contrast to our 'word of caution' on p.124, thinking about the causes of 'mental health problems' can sometimes get rid of the 'problem' all by itself.

One of the dilemmas in all of this was illustrated by the research (which we wrote about in Chapter 7) showing that, when we are depressed, we sometimes see the world more accurately than when we are happy. So, to some extent, you have to decide for yourself whether it is better to be happy or wise.

Of course, people sometimes need to do something more than just accept that most people would have reacted the way they did under the same circumstances. In that case, a good place to start is having an understanding of which factors, in the world around them and in their own minds, have contributed and which ones may still be contributing. Then decide what course of action to take. Professionals need to be aware of these possibilities too – if the cause is an environmental factor, it will probably be worthwhile trying to change the environment, or trying to avoid certain aspects of it.

Thinking about the causes of mental health problems may not only help us accept or change ourselves; we could also end up doing our own small bit, one way or another, to change that small part of the world we have some influence over, to reduce that cause of distress for everyone. We imagine many readers will be already doing that.

It would have been frustrating for readers if we'd said this at the outset, but we hope this book has provided more questions than answers. Acknowledging how little we collectively know is the first step towards finding out something worth saying about the causes of mental health problems.

And so we end with one more question regarding the causes of psychological distress. Given the high numbers of people experiencing mental health problems of some kind (we are told that one in four of us will do so at some point in our lives (WHO, 2001)), is it time we started to think about the role the societies we live in play in causing this huge and apparently ever-increasing amount of human unhappiness and distress, and what we can all do to prevent them?

George Albee put it this way:

> Psychologists must join with persons who reject racism, sexism, colonialism, and exploitation and must find ways to redistribute social power and to increase social justice. Primary prevention research inevitably will make clear the relationship between social pathology and psychopathology and then will work to change social and political structures in

the interests of social justice. It is as simple and as difficult as that! (Albee, 1996, p.113)

Richard Wilkinson and Kate Pickett, authors of *The Spirit Level*, put it like this (referring to the graphs reproduced in Chapter 6, showing that prevalence of mental illness is more prevalent in more unequal affluent societies):

The solution to problems caused by inequality is not mass psychotherapy aimed at making everyone less vulnerable. The best way of responding to the harm done by high levels of inequality would be to reduce the inequality itself. Rather than requiring anti-anxiety drugs in the water supply or mass psychotherapy, what is most exciting about the picture we present is that it shows that reducing inequality would increase the wellbeing and quality of life for all of us. (2009, p.33)

But the final, final words of course must go to Pete Sanders, my dear friend and collaborator:

Thinking and feeling are not sufficient. *Being* is not enough – *doing* completes the picture. When separated, not only are being and doing both the poorer, but so is the whole human race, connected as we are. To be whole political entities, we each need to act, whether in our individual domain of influence or in community with others. It doesn't matter what we do, as long as our doing remains true to our values, but *doing* is one of the ways we can reconnect with our experience, each other and the world. (Sanders, 2006b, p.315)

References

Ainsworth, M.D.S. & Bell, S.M. (1970). Attachment, exploration, and separation: Illustrated by the behavior of one-year-olds in a strange situation. *Child Development, 41*, 49–67.

Albee, G. (1985). The argument for primary prevention. *Journal of Primary Prevention, 5*, 213–219.

Albee, G. (1996). Revolutions and counter-revolutions in prevention. *American Psychologist, 51*, 1130–1133.

Alexander, F. & Selesnick, S. (1996). *The history of psychiatric thought and practice from prehistoric times to the present.* Harper & Row.

Alloy, L. & Abramson, L. (1979). Judgement of contingency in depressed and non-depressed students: Sadder but wiser? *Journal of Experimental Psychology: General, 108*(4), 441–485.

American Psychiatric Association (APA). (1987). *The diagnostic and statistical manual of mental disorders* (3rd ed. rev.), (DSM-III-TR). APA.

American Psychiatric Association (APA). (2000). *The diagnostic and statistical manual of mental disorders* (4th ed. rev.), (DSM-IV-TR). APA.

American Psychiatric Association (APA). (2013). *The diagnostic and statistical manual of mental disorders* (5th ed.), (DSM-5). APA.

Angermeyer, M. & Dietrich, S. (2006). Public beliefs about and attitudes towards people with mental illness: A review of population studies. *Acta Psychiatrica Scandinavica, 113*(3), 163–179.

Angermeyer, M., Klusmann, D. & Walpuski, O. (1988). The causes of functional psychoses as seen by patients and their relatives. II: The relatives' point of view. *European Archives of Psychiatry and Neurological Sciences, 238*(1), 55–61.

Appignanesi, R. & Zarate, O. (2003). *Freud for beginners.* Pantheon.

Bandura, A. (1977). *Social learning theory.* Prentice Hall.

Barry, M. & Greene, S. (1992). Implicit models of mental disorder. *Irish Journal of Psychology, 13*(2), 141–160.

Bebbington, P.E., Bhugra, D., Brugha, T., Singleton, N., Farrell, M., Jenkins, R., Lewis, G. & Meltzer, H. (2004). Psychosis, victimization and childhood disadvantage: Evidence from the second British National Survey of Psychiatric Morbidity. *British Journal of Psychiatry, 185,* 220–226.

Bentall, R.P. (2004). Abandoning the concept of schizophrenia. In J. Read, L.R. Mosher & R.P. Bentall (Eds.), *Models of madness* (pp.196–208). Routledge.

Bentall, R.P. (2009). *Doctoring the mind: Why psychiatric treatments fail.* Penguin.

Blehar, M.C. & Rosenthal, N.E. (1989). Seasonal affective disorders and phototherapy. Report of a National Institute of Mental Health-sponsored workshop. *Archives of General Psychiatry, 46*(5), 469–474.

Bourdieu, P. (1977). *Outline of a theory of practice.* Cambridge University Press.

Bowlby, J. (1951). *Child care and the growth of love.* Penguin.

Bowlby, J. (1969). *Attachment and loss. Vol 1: Attachment.* Pimlico.

Bowlby, J. (1973). *Attachment and Loss. Vol 2: Separation: Anger and anxiety.* Pimlico.

Bowlby, J. (1980). *Attachment and Loss. Vol 3: Loss: Sadness and depression.* Hogarth Press/ Institute of Psychoanalysis.

Boyle, M. & Johnstone, L. (2020). *A straight talking introduction to the Power Threat Meaning Framework: An alternative to psychiatric diagnosis.* PCCS Books.

British Psychological Society (BPS). (2013). *Classification of behaviour and experience in relation to functional psychiatric diagnoses: Time for a paradigm shift.* British Psychological Society.

Brody, D.J. & Gu, Q. (2020). *Antidepressant use among adults: United States, 2015–2018.* Data Brief 377. National Centre for Health Statistics.

Bullimore, P. (2010). My personal experience of psychosis. *Psychosis: Psychological, Social and Integrative Approaches, 2*(2), 173–177.

Burton, R. (1621/1961). *The anatomy of melancholy: Volume 2.* Dent.

Cahalan, S. (2019). *The great pretender.* Canongate Books.

Carter, L., Read, J., Pyle, M. & Morrison, A. (2017). The impact of causal explanations on outcome in people experiencing psychosis: A systematic review. *Clinical Psychology & Psychotherapy, 24*(2), 332–347.

Cash, A. (2021). *Psychology for dummies*. Wiley.

Cervone, D. & Pervin, L. (2008). *Personality: Theory and research* (10th ed.). Wiley.

Champagne, F. & Curley, J. (2009). Epigenetic mechanisms mediating the long-term effects of maternal care on development. *Neuroscience and Biobehavioral Reviews, 33*(4), 593–600.

Clements, J. & Davies, E. (2013). Prevention of psychosis: Creating societies where more people flourish. In J. Read & J. Dillon (Eds.), *Models of madness* (pp.295–304). Routledge.

Cooper, M., Watson, J.C. & Hölldampf, D. (2010). *Person-centered and experiential therapies work*. PCCS Books.

Copeland, J.R.M., Cooper, J.E., Kendell, R.E. & Gourlay, A.J. (1971). Differences in usage of diagnostic labels amongst psychiatrists in the British Isles. *British Journal of Psychiatry, 118*(547), 629–640.

Cosgrove, L. & Krimsky, S. (2012). A comparison of DSM-IV and DSM-5 panel members' financial associations with industry: A pernicious problem persists. *PLoS Medicine, 9*(3): e1001190. https://doi.org/10.1371/journal.pmed.1001190

Cozolino, L., Goldstein, M., Nuechterlein, W., West, K. & Snyder, K. (1988). The impact of education about schizophrenia on relatives varying in expressed emotion. *Schizophrenia Bulletin, 14*(4), 675–687.

Cromby, J., Harper, D. & Reavey, P. (2013a). History. In J. Cromby, D. Harper & P. Reavey, *Psychology, mental health and distress* (pp.19–51). Palgrave MacMillan.

Cromby, J., Harper, D. & Reavey, P. (2013b). Biology. In J. Cromby, D. Harper & P. Reavey, *Psychology, mental health and distress* (pp.75–100). Palgrave MacMillan.

Cromby, J., Harper, D. & Reavey, P. (2013c). Diagnosis and formulation. In J. Cromby, D. Harper & P. Reavey, *Psychology, mental health and distress* (pp.101–117). Palgrave MacMillan.

Cromby, J., Harper, D. & Reavey, P. (2013d). Causal influences. In J. Cromby, D. Harper & P. Reavey, *Psychology, mental health and distress* (pp.118–138). Palgrave MacMillan.

Cromby, J., Harper, D. & Reavey, P. (2013e). Interventions. In J. Cromby, D. Harper & P. Reavey, *Psychology, mental health and distress* (pp.158–190). Palgrave MacMillan.

Davies, E. & Burdett, J. (2004). Preventing 'schizophrenia': Creating the conditions for saner societies. In J. Read, L. Mosher & R. Bentall (Eds.), *Models of madness* (pp.271–282). Routledge.

Davies, E., Read, J. & Shevlin, M. (2021). The impact of adverse childhood experiences and recent life events on anxiety and quality of life in university students. *Higher Education.* https://doi.org/10.1007/s10734-021-00774-9

Davies, J. (2013). *Cracked: Why psychiatry is doing more harm than good.* Icon Books.

Davies, J. (2021). *Sedated. How modern capitalism created our mental health crisis.* Atlantic Books.

Davies, J. (2022, August 5). Calling someone 'anti-psychiatry' is not an argument. *Mad in the UK.* www.madintheuk.com/2022/08/anti-psychiatry-argument-criticisms

De Wattigner, S. & Read, J. (2009). The pharmaceutical industry and the internet: Are drug company funded depression websites biased? *Journal of Mental Health, 18*(6), 476–485.

Dillon, J. (2010). The tale of an ordinary little girl. *Psychosis: Psychological, Social and Integrative Approaches, 2*(1), 79–83.

Dilsaver, S.C., Wetterberg, L., Blehar, M.C. & Rosenthal, N.E. (1990). Onset of winter depression earlier than generally thought? *Journal of Clinical Psychiatry, 51*(6), 258.

Ducey, C. & Simon, B. (1975). Ancient Greece and Rome. In J. G. Howells (Ed.), *World history of psychiatry* (pp.1–38). Brunner/Mazel.

Eaton, W. (1980). A formal theory of selection for schizophrenia. *American Journal of Sociology, 86(*1), 149–158.

Felitti, V., Anda, R., Nordenberg, D., Williamson, D., Spitz, A., Edwards, V., Koss, M. & Marks, J. (1998). Adverse childhood experiences. *American Journal of Preventive Medicine, 14(*4), 245–258.

Fonagy, P., Gyorgy, G., Jurist, E.L. & Target, M. (2004). *Affect regulation, mentalization and the development of self.* Karnac.

Fortney, J., Rushton, G., Wood, S., Zhang, L., Xu, S., Dong, F. & Rost, K. (2007). Community-level risk factors for depression hospitalizations. *Administration and Policy in Mental Health and Mental Health Services Research, 34(*4), 343–352.

Foucault, M. (1967). *Madness and civilisation.* Random House.

Foucault, M. (2006). *A history of madness.* (J. Khalfa, Trans.). Routledge.

Frances, A. (2012, December 12). DSM-5 in distress. *Psychology Today.* www.psychologytoday.com/blog/dsm5-in-distress/201212/dsm-5-is-guide-not-bible-ignore-its-ten-worst-changes

Freud, S. (2010). *The interpretation of dreams.* (J. Moussaieff Masson, (Ed.), A.A. Brill (Trans.).) Sterling.

Freud, S., Strachey, J., Freud, A., Rothgeb, C.L. & Richards, A. (1953–1974). *The standard edition of the complete psychological works of Sigmund Freud.* Hogarth Press.

Friedli, L. & Stearn, R. (2015). Positive affect as coercive strategy: Conditionality, activation and the role of psychology in UK government workfare programmes. *Medical Humanities, 41*(1), 40–47.

Fromm, E. (1956). *The art of loving.* Harper & Brothers.

Fromm, E. (2002). *The sane society* (2nd ed.). Routledge.

Fromm, E. (2003). *Man for himself, an inquiry into the psychology of ethics.* Routledge.

Fromm-Reichmann, F. (1989). *Psychoanalysis and psychosis.* International Universities Press.

Furnham, A. & Bower, P. (1992). A comparison of academic and lay theories of schizophrenia. *British Journal of Psychiatry, 161*, 201–210.

Furnham, A. & Rees, J. (1988). Lay theories of schizophrenia. *International Journal of Social Psychiatry, 34*, 212–220.

Geekie, J. & Read, J. (2009). *Making sense of madness: Contesting the meaning of schizophrenia.* Routledge.

Geekie, J., Randal, P., Lampshire, D. & Read, J. (2011). *Experiencing psychosis.* Routledge.

Gosden, L. & Krimsky S. (2012). A comparison of DSM-IV and DSM-5 panel members' financial associations with industry: A pernicious problem persists. *PLoS Med, 9*(3) e1001190

Greenberg, J. (1964). *I never promised you a rose garden.* Holt, Rinehart & Winston.

Griffiths, A. (2019). Reflections on using the Power Threat Meaning Framework in peer-led systems. *Clinical Psychology Forum, 313*, 25–32.

Haaga, D. & Beck, A. (1995). Perspectives on depressive realism. *Behaviour Research and Therapy, 33*(1), 41–48.

Hahn, P. (2019). *Madness and genetic determinism.* Palgrave MacMillan.

Hall, W. & Degenhardt, L. (2000). Cannabis use and psychosis: A review of clinical and epidemiological evidence. *Australian and New Zealand Journal of Psychiatry, 34*(1), 26–34.

Hamilton, S. (2008). Schizophrenia candidate genes: Are we really coming up blank? *American Journal of Psychiatry, 165*(4), 420–423.

Hanh Le Quan-Bui, K., Plaisant, O., Leboyer, M., Gay, C., Kamal, L., Devynck, M.-A. & Meyer, P. (1984). Reduced platelet serotonin in depression. *Psychiatry Research, 13*(2), 129–139.

Harrison G., Gunnell, D., Glazebrook, C., Page, K. & Kwiecinski, R. (2001). Association between schizophrenia and social inequality at birth. *British Journal of Psychiatry, 179*, 346–350.

Harrop, C.E. & Trower, P. (2001). Why does schizophrenia develop at late adolescence? *Clinical Psychology Review, 21*(2), 241–265.

Haslam, N., Bastian, B., Bain, P. & Kashima, Y. (2006). Psychological essentialism, implicit theories, and intergroup relations. *Group Processes & Intergroup Relations, 9*, 63–76.

Heald, A., Stedman, M., Davies M., Livingston, M., Taylor, D. & Gadsby, R. (2020). Antidepressant prescribing in England: Patterns and costs. *Primary Care Companion for CNS Disorders, 22*, 19m02552.

Healy, D. & Thase, M.E. (2003). Is academic psychiatry for sale? *British Journal of Psychiatry, 182*(5), 388–391.

Herron, W.G., Schultz, C.L. & Welt, A.G. (1992). A comparison of 16 systems to diagnose schizophrenia. *Journal of Clinical Psychology, 48*(6), 711–721.

Hills, P. & Pake, M. (2016). *Cognitive psychology for dummies*. Wiley.

Hippocrates. (1931). *Sacred heart.* (W. Jones, Trans.). Heinemann.

Hollingshead, A.B. & Redlich, F.C. (1954). Schizophrenia and social structure. *American Journal of Psychiatry, 110*, 695–701.

Holzinger, A., Loffler, W., Muller, P., Priebe, S. & Angermeyer, M. (2002). Subjective illness theory and antipsychotic medication compliance by patients with schizophrenia. *Journal of Nervous & Mental Disease, 190*(9), 597–603.

Janowsky, D.S. & Risch, S.C. (1984). Adrenergic-cholinergic balance and affective disorders: A review of clinical evidence and therapeutic implications. *Psychiatric Hospital, 15*, 163–171.

Janssen, I., Hanssen, M., Bak, M., Bijl, R., De Graaf, R., Vollebergh, W., McKenzie, K. & van Os, J. (2003). Discrimination and delusional ideation. *British Journal of Psychiatry, 182*, 71–76.

Jenkins, T.A., Nguyen, J.C.D., Polgaze, K.E. & Bertrand, P.P. (2016). Influence of tryptophan and serotonin on mood and cognition with a possible role of the gut-brain axis. *Nutrients, 8*(1), 56. https://doi.org/10.3390/nu8010056

Johnson, R., Antonaccio, O., Botchkovar, E. & Hobfoll, S. (2022). War trauma and PTSD in Ukraine's civilian population. *Social Psychiatry and Psychiatric Epidemiology, 57*(1), 1807–1816.

Johnstone, L. (2022). *A straight-talking introduction to psychiatric diagnoses* (2nd ed.). PCCS Books.

Johnstone, L. & Boyle, M., with Cromby, J., Dillon, J., Harper, D., Kinderman, P., Longden, E., Pilgrim, D. & Read, J. (2018). *The Power Threat Meaning*

Framework: Towards the identification of patterns in emotional distress, unusual experiences and troubled or troubling behaviour, as an alternative to functional psychiatric diagnosis. British Psychological Society.

Joint Commission on Mental Illness and Health. (1961). *Action for mental health*. Basic Books.

Joseph, J. (2005). T*he missing gene: Psychiatry, heredity and the fruitless search for genes.* Algora.

Joseph, J. (2022a, August 31). Major depression: the 'chemical imbalance' pillar is crumbling. Is the genetics pillar next? *Mad in America.* www.madinamerica.com/2022/08/depression-genetics-pillar/

Joseph, J. (2022b). *Schizophrenia and genetics: The end of an illusion.* Routledge.

Joshi S., Mooney S., Rundle A., Quinn J., Beard J. & Cerdá, M. (2017). Pathways from neighborhood poverty to depression among older adults. *Health and Place, 43*, 138–143.

Jung, C. (1961/1997). *Man and his symbols.* Bantam Doubleday Dell.

Kakaje, A., Al Zohbi, R. & Hosam Aldeen, O. (2021). Mental disorder and PTSD in Syria during wartime: A nationwide crisis. *BMC Psychiatry, 21*. https://doi.org/10.1186/s12888-020-03002-3

Karanci, A. (1995). Caregivers of Turkish schizophrenic patients: Causal attributions, burdens and attitudes to help from the health professions. *Social Psychiatry and Psychiatric Epidemiology, 30*(6), 261–268.

Khalifeh, H., Moran, P., Borschmann, R., Dean, K., Hart, C., Hogg, J., Osborn, D., Johnson, S. & Howard, L. (2015). Domestic and sexual violence against patients with severe mental illness. *Psychological Medicine, 45*(4), 875–886. https://doi.org/10.1017/S0033291714001962

Kirsch, I., Deacon, B., Huedo-Medina, T., Scoboria, A., Moore, T. & Johnson, B. (2008). Initial severity and antidepressant benefits: A meta-analysis of data submitted to the Food and Drug Administration. *PLOS Medicine, 5*, 260–268.

Kirschenbaum, H. (2007). *The life and work of Carl Rogers.* PCCS Books.

Klein, D., Lewinsohn, P., Seeley, R. & Rohde, P. (2001). A family study of major depressive disorder in a community sample of adolescents. *Archives of General Psychiatry, 58*(1), 13–20.

Kohn, M. (1976). The interaction of social class and other factors in the etiology of schizophrenia. *American Journal of Psychiatry, 133*(2), 177–180.

Kraemer, M. & Sprenger, M. (1486/1941). *Malleus maleficarum.* (J. Summer, Trans.). Pushkin.

Kutchins, H. & Kirk, S.A. (1999). *Making us crazy: DSM – The psychiatric bible and the creation of mental disorders.* Constable.

Kvaale, E.P., Gottdiener, W. & Haslam, N. (2013a). Biogenetic explanations and stigma: A meta-analytic review of associations among laypeople. *Social Science and Medicine, 96,* 95–103.

Kvaale, E.P., Gottdiener, W.& Haslam, N. (2013b). The 'side effects' of medicalization: A meta-analytic review of how bio-genetic explanations affect stigma. *Clinical Psychology Review, 33*(6), 782–794.

Larkin, W. & Morrison, A. (Eds.). (2006). *Trauma and psychosis: New directions for theory and therapy.* Routledge.

Larkin, W. & Read, J. (2008). Childhood trauma and psychosis: Evidence, pathways, and implications. *Journal of Postgraduate Medicine, 54*(4), 284–290.

Larkings, J.S. & Brown, P.M. (2018). Do biogenetic causal beliefs reduce mental illness stigma in people with mental illness and in mental health professionals? A systematic review. *International Journal of Mental Health Nursing, 27*(3), 928–941.

Lebowitz, M. & Ahn, W. (2014). Effects of biological explanations for mental disorders on clinicians' empathy. *Proceedings of the National Academy of Science of the USA, 111*(50), 17786–17790.

Lee, C., Oliffe, J.L., Kelly, M.T. & Ferlatte, O. (2017). Depression and suicidality in gay men: Implications for health care providers. *American Journal of Men's Health, 11*(4), 910–919.

Liu, Q., He, H., Yang, J., Feng, X., Zhao, F. & Lyu, J. (2020). Changes in the global burden of depression from 1990 to 2017: Findings from the Global Burden of Disease study. *Journal of Psychiatric Research, 126,* 134–140.

Longden, E. & Read, J. (2017). People with problems, not patients with illnesses: Using psychosocial frameworks to reduce the stigma of psychosis. *Israel Journal of Psychiatry and Related Sciences, 54*(1), 24–28.

Magliano, L., De Rosa, C., Fiorillo, A., Malangone, C., Guarneri, M., Marasco, C., Maj, M. & Working Group of the Italian National Study. (2004). Beliefs of psychiatric nurses about schizophrenia: A comparison with patients' relatives and psychiatrists. *International Journal of Social Psychiatry, 50*(4), 319–330.

Magliano, L., Fiorillo, A., Del Vecchio, H., Malangone, C., De Rosa, C., Bachelet, C.,Truglia, E., D'Ambrogio, R., Pizzale, F., Veltro, F., Zanus, P., Pioli, R. & Maj, M. (2009). What people with schizophrenia think about the causes of their disorder. *Epidemiology and Psychiatric Sciences, 18*(1), 48–53.

Martinez, A.G., Piff, P.K., Mendoza-Denton, R. & Hinshaw, S.P. (2011). The power of a label: Mental illness diagnoses, ascribed humanity, and social rejection. *Journal of Social and Clinical Psychology, 30*(1), 1–23.

Masson, J. (1984). *The assault on truth: Freud and the seduction theory.* Farrar, Straus & Giroux.

McBride, O., Murphy, J., Shevlin, M., Givson-Miller, J., Hartman, T.K., Hyland, P., Levita, L., Mason, L., Martinez, A.P., McKay, R., Va Stocks, T., Bennett, K.M., Valières, F., Karatzias, T., Valiente, C., Vazquez, C. & Bentall, R. (2021). Monitoring the psychological, social, and economic impact of the COVID-19 pandemic in the population. *International Journal of Methods in Psychiatric Research, 30*(1) e1861.

McCabe, R. & Priebe, S. (2004). Explanatory models of illness in schizophrenia: Comparison of four ethnic groups. *British Journal of Psychiatry, 185,* 25–30.

McCartney, G., Hart, C. & Watt, G. (2013). How can socioeconomic inequalities in hospital admissions be explained? A cohort study. *BMJ Open, 3,* e002433.

McGill, C., Falloon, I., Boyd, J. & Wood-Siverio, C. (1983). Family educational intervention in the treatment of schizophrenia. *Hospital & Community Psychiatry, 34*(10) 934–938.

Michelet, J. (1939). *Satanism and witchcraft.* Citadel.

Miller, N. (1975). Israel and the Jews. In J. Howells (Ed.), *World history of psychiatry* (pp.528–546). Brunner/Mazel.

Moncrieff, J. (2020). *A straight talking introduction to psychiatric drugs: The truth about how they work and how to come off them* (2nd ed.). PCCS Books.

Moncrieff, J., Cooper, R.E., Stockmann. T., Amendola, S., Hengartner, M.P. & Horowitz, M.A. (2022). The serotonin theory of depression: A systematic umbrella review of the evidence. *Molecular Psychiatry.* https://doi.org/10.1038/s41380-022-01661-0. Epub ahead of print. PMID: 35854107.

Morgan, C., Kirkbride, J., Leff, J., Craig, T., Hutchinson, G., McKenzie, K., Morgan, K., Dazzan, P., Doody, G.A., Jones, P., Murray, R. & Fearon, P. (2007). Parental separation, loss and psychosis in different ethnic groups: A case-control study. *Psychological Medicine, 37*(4), 495–503.

Mosher, L.R., Gosden, R. & Beder, S. (2013). Drug companies and schizophrenia: Unbridled capitalism meets madness. In J. Read & J. Dillon (Eds.), *Models of madness* (2nd ed.) (pp.125–140). Routledge.

Moskowitz, A., Dorahy, M.J. & Schafer, I. (Eds.). (2019). *Psychosis, trauma and dissociation: Evolving perspectives on severe psychopathology* (2nd ed.). Wiley.

Moynihan, R. & Cassels, A. (2005). *Selling sickness: How the world's biggest pharmaceutical companies are turning us all into patients.* Nation Books.

Mullen, P., Martin, J., Anderson, J., Romans, S. & Herbison, G. (1993). Childhood sexual abuse and mental health in adult life. *British Journal of Psychiatry, 163*(6), 721–732.

Murray, R.M. (2017). Mistakes I have made in my research career. *Schizophrenia Bulletin, 43*(2), 253–256.

OECD. (2021, June 28). OECD health statistics 2021. *Pharmaceutical Market.* https://stats.oecd.org/Index.aspx?DataSetCode=HEALTH_PHMC

Pariante, C. (2022). Depression is both psychosocial and biological; antidepressants are both effective and in need of improvement; psychiatrists are both caring human beings and doctors who prescribe medications. Can we all agree on this? A commentary on 'Read & Moncrieff – depression: Why drugs and electricity are not the answer'. *Psychological Medicine*, 1–3. https://doi.org/10.1017/S0033291722000770

Pedersen, C. & Mortensen, P. (2001). Urbanization and schizophrenia. *Schizophrenia Research, S41*, 65–66.

Pilkington, P.D., Reavley, N.J. & Jorm, A.F. (2013). The Australian public's beliefs about the causes of depression. *Journal of Affective Disorders, 150*(2), 356–362.

Pistrang, N. & Barker, C. (1992). Clients' beliefs about psychological problems. *Counselling Psychology Quarterly, 5*(4), 325–335.

Plato. (1904). *Timaeus.* (R. Bury, Trans.). Harvard University Press.

Porter, R. (2002). *Madness: A brief history*. Oxford University Press.

Rampello, L., Nicoletti, F. & Nicoletti, F. (2000). Dopamine and depression: Therapeutic implications. *CNS Drugs, 13*, 35–45.

Read, J. (2010). Can poverty drive you mad? 'Schizophrenia', socioeconomic status and the case for primary prevention. *New Zealand Journal of Psychology, 39*(2), 7–19.

Read, J. (2013a). A history of madness. In J. Read & J. Dillon (Eds.), *Models of madness* (pp.9–19). Routledge.

Read, J. (2013b). Biological psychiatry's lost cause: The 'schizophrenic brain. In J. Read & J. Dillon (Eds.), *Models of madness* (pp.62–71). Routledge.

Read, J. (2020). Bad things happen and can drive you crazy: The causal beliefs of 701 people taking antipsychotics. *Psychiatry Research, 285*, 112754.

Read, J. (2021, August 11). Understanding our psychological reactions to COVID. *Psychology Today.* https://www.psychologytoday.com/gb/blog/psychiatry-through-the-looking-glass/202108/understanding-our-psychological-reactions-covid

Read, J. & Beavan, V, (2013). Gender and psychosis. In J. Read & J. Dillon (Eds.), *Models of madness* (pp.210-219). Routledge.

Read, J. & Cain, A. (2013). A literature review and meta-analysis of drug company funded mental health websites. *Acta Psychiatrica Scandinavica, 128*(6), 422–433.

Read, J. & Gumley, A. (2008). Can attachment theory help explain the relationship between childhood adversity and psychosis? *Attachment: New Directions in Psychotherapy and Relational Psychoanalysis, 2,* 1–35.

Read, J. & Harper, D. (2022). The Power Threat Meaning Framework: Addressing adversity, challenging prejudice and stigma and transforming services. *Journal of Constructivist Psychology, 35*(1), 54–67.

Read, J. & Magliano, L. (2011). The subjective experience and beliefs of relatives of people who experience psychosis. In J. Geekie, P. Randal, D. Lampshire & J. Read, (Eds.), *Experiencing psychosis* (pp.207–216). Routledge.

Read, J. & Masson, J. (2013). Genetics, eugenics and mass murder. In J. Read & J. Dillon (Eds.). *Models of madness* (pp.34–46). Routledge.

Read, J. & Masson J. (2022). Biological psychiatry and the mass murder of 'schizophrenics': From denial to inspirational alternative. *Ethical Human Psychology and Psychiatry,* doi:10:1891/EHPP-2021-0006.

Read, J. & Moncrieff, J. (2022). Depression: Why drugs and electricity are not the answer. *Psychological Medicine, 52*(8), 1402–1410.

Read, J., Agar, K., Barker-Collo, S., Davies, E. & Moskowitz, A. (2001b). Assessing suicidality in adults: Integrating childhood trauma as a major risk factor. *Professional Psychology: Research and Practice, 32,* 367–372.

Read, J., Bentall, R.P. & Fosse, R. (2009). Time to abandon the bio-bio-bio model of psychosis: Exploring the epigenetic and psychological mechanisms by which adverse life events lead to psychotic symptoms. *Epidemiologia e Psichiatria Sociale, 18*(4), 299–310.

Read, J., Cartwright, C., Gibson, K., Shiels, C., Haslam, N. (2014b). Beliefs of people taking antidepressants about causes of depression and reasons for increased prescribing rates. *Journal of Affective Disorders, 168,* 236–242.

Read, J., Fink, P., Rudegeair, T., Felitti, V. & Whitfield, C. (2008). Child maltreatment and psychosis: A return to a genuinely integrated bio-psycho-social model. *Clinical Schizophrenia and Related Psychoses, 7,* 235–254.

Read, J., Fosse, R., Moskowitz, A. & Perry, B. (2014a). The traumagenic neurodevelopmental model of psychosis revisited. *Neuropsychiatry, 4*(1), 65–79.

Read, J., Harrop, C., Geekie, J., Renton, J. & Cunliffe, S. (2021). A second independent audit of ECT in England: Usage, demographics, consent, and adherence to guidelines and legislation in 2019. *Psychology and Psychotherapy: Theory, Research and Practice, 94*(3), 603–619

Read, J., Haslam N. & Magliano, L. (2013a). Prejudice, stigma and 'schizophrenia': The role of bio-genetic ideology. In J. Read & J. Dillon (Eds.), *Models of madness* (pp.157–177). Routledge.

Read, J., Haslam, N., Sayce, L. & Davies, E. (2006). Prejudice and schizophrenia: A review of the 'Mental illness is an illness like any other' approach. *Acta Psychiatrica Scandinavica, 114*(5), 303-318.

Read, J., Johnstone, L. & Taitimu, M. (2013c). Psychosis, poverty and ethnicity. Poverty, ethnicity and gender. In J. Read & J. Dillon (Eds.), *Models of madness* (2nd ed), (pp.191-209). Routledge.

Read, J., Kirsch, I. & Mcgrath, L. (2019). Electroconvulsive therapy for depression: A review of the quality of ECT vs sham ECT trials and meta-analyses. *Ethical Human Psychiatry and Psychology, 21*(2), 64-103.

Read, J., Magliano, M. & Beavan, V. (2013b). Public beliefs about the causes of 'schizophrenia': Bad things happen and can drive you crazy. In J. Read & J. Dillon (Eds.), *Models of madness* (pp.143-156). Routledge.

Read, J., Perry, B., Moskowitz, A. & Connolly, J. (2001a). The contribution of early traumatic events to schizophrenia in some patients: A traumagenic neurodevelopmental model. *Psychiatry: Interpersonal and Biological Processes, 64*(4), 319-345.

Read, J., van Os, J., Morrison, A. & Ross, C. (2005). Childhood trauma, psychosis and schizophrenia: A literature review with theoretical and clinical implications. *Acta Psychiatrica Scandinavica, 112*(5), 330-350.

Reil, J. (1803). *Rhapsodien uber die anwendung der psychischen curmethode auf geisteszerruttungen.* Curt.

Rogers, C.R. (1951). *Client-centered therapy: Its current practice, implications, and theory.* Constable.

Rogers, D. & Pilgrim, D. (1997). The contribution of lay knowledge to the understanding and promotion of mental health. *Journal of Mental Health, 6*(1), 23-36.

Romme, M., Escher, S., Dillon, J., Corstens, D. & Morris, M. (Eds.). (2009). *Living with voices: 50 stories of recovery.* PCCS Books.

Rose, S. (2005). *The 21st century brain: Explaining, mending and manipulating the mind.* Jonathan Cape.

Rosen, G. (1964). *Madness in society.* University of Chicago Press.

Rosenhan, D. (1975). On being sane in insane places. *Science, 179*(4070), 250-258.

Ross, C. (2020). *The genetics of schizophrenia.* Manitou Communications.

Ryan, C., Huebner, D., Diaz, R.M. & Sanchez, J. (2009). Family rejection as a predictor of negative health outcomes in white and Latino lesbian, gay, and bisexual young adults. *Pediatrics, 123*(1), 346-352.

Sagayadevan, V., Lau, Y.W., Zhang, Y., Jeyagurunathan, A., Shafie, S., Chang, S., Chong, S.A. & Subramaniam, M. (2020). Caregivers' causal attributions of their relatives' mental illness and the association with stigma. *Transcultural Psychiatry, 57*(3), 421–431.

Sampson, L., Ettman, C.K. & Galea, S. (2020). Urbanization, urbanicity, and depression: A review of the recent global literature. *Current Opinion in Psychiatry, 33*(3), 233–244.

Sanders, A., Duan, J., Levinson, D., Shi, J., He, D., Hou, C., Burrell, G.J., Rice, J.P., Nertney, D.A., Olincy, A., Rozic, P., Vinogradov, S., Buccola, N.G., Mowry, B.J., Freeman, R., Amin, F., Black, D.W., Silverman, J.M., Byerley, W.F. ... Gejman, P.V. (2008). No significant association of 14 candidate genes with schizophrenia in a large European ancestry sample: Implications for psychiatric genetics. *American Journal of Psychiatry, 165*(4), 497–506.

Sanders, P. (2006a). *The person-centred counselling primer*. PCCS Books.

Sanders, P. (2006b). Concluding remarks. In G. Proctor, M. Cooper, P. Sanders & B. Malcolm, *Politicising the person-centred approach: An agenda for social change* (pp.313–315). PCCS Books.

Schatzberg, A. (2002). Brain imaging in affective disorders: More questions about causes versus effects. *American Journal of Psychiatry, 159*(11), 1807–1808.

Schlenger, W.E., Corry, N.H., Williams, C.S., Kulka, R.A., Mulvaney-Day, N., DeBakey, S., Murphy, C.M. & Marmar, C.R. (2015). A prospective study of mortality and trauma-related risk factors among a nationally representative sample of Vietnam veterans. *American Journal of Epidemiology, 182*(12), 980–990.

Scull, A. (1981). Moral treatment reconsidered. In A. Scull (Ed.), *Madhouses, mad-doctors and madmen* (pp.105–188). University of Philadelphia.

Sharfstein, S. (2005). Big Pharma and American psychiatry: The good, the bad and the ugly. *Psychiatric News, 40*(16), 3.

Shevlin, M., Butter, S., McBride, O., Murphy, J., Gibson-Miller, J., Hartman, T.K., Levita, L., Mason, L., Martinez, A.P., McKay, R., Stocks, T.V.A., Bennett, K., Hyland, P. & Bentall, R. (2021). Refuting the myth of a 'tsunami' of mental ill-health in populations affected by COVID-19: Evidence that response to the pandemic is heterogeneous, not homogeneous. *Psychological Medicine*, 1–9.

Shevlin, M., Dorahy, M. & Adamson, G. (2007). Childhood traumas and hallucinations: An analysis of the National Comorbidity Survey. *Journal of Psychiatric Research, 41*(3–4), 222–228.

Shevlin, M., McBride, O., Murphy, J., Gibson Miller, J., Hartman, T.K., Levita, L., Mason, L., Martinez, A.P., McKay, R., Stocks, T.V.A., Bennett, K.M., Hyland, P., Karatzias, T. & Bentall, R. (2020). Anxiety, depression, traumatic stress and COVID-19-related anxiety in the UK general population during the COVID-19 pandemic. *British Journal of Psychiatry Open, 6*(6), e125.

Shevlin, M., Murphy, J., Houston, J.E. & Adamson, G. (2009). Childhood sexual abuse, early cannabis use and psychosis: Testing the effects of different temporal orderings based on the National Comorbidity Survey. *Psychosis, 1*(1), 19–28.

Shooter, M. (2005). Dancing with the devil? A personal view of psychiatry's relationship with the pharmaceutical industry. *Psychiatric Bulletin, 29*(3), 81–83.

Skinner, B.F. (1948). *Walden two*. Hackett.

Slater, L. (2004). *Opening Skinner's box: Great psychological experiments of the twentieth century*. Norton.

Srinivasan, T.N. & Thara, R. (2001). Beliefs about causation of schizophrenia: Do Indian families believe in supernatural causes? *Social Psychiatry and Psychiatric Epidemiology, 36*(3), 134–140.

Stansfield, S.A., Clark, C., Rodgers, B., Caldwell, T. & Power, C. (2008). Childhood and adulthood socio-economic position and midlife depressive and anxiety disorders. *British Journal of Psychiatry, 192*(2), 152–153.

Storr, A. (2001). *Freud: A very short introduction*. Oxford University Press.

Sullivan, H.S. (1953). *The interpersonal theory of psychiatry*. W.W. Norton & Co.

Suokas, K., Koivisto, A. & Hakulinen, C. (2019). Association of income with the incidence rates of first psychiatric hospital admission rates in Finland, 1996–2014. *JAMA Psychiatry, 77*(3), 274–284.

Sweeney, A., Clement, S., Filson, B. & Kennedy, A. (2016). Trauma-informed mental healthcare in the UK: What is it and how can we further its development? *Mental Health Review Journal, 21*(3), 174–192.

Taylor, J. (2022). *Sexy but psycho: How the patriarchy uses women's trauma against them*. Constable.

Taylor, S., Annand, F., Burkinshaw, P., Greaves, F., Kelleher, M., Knight, J., Perkins C, Tran, A., White, M. & Marsden J. (2019). *Dependence and withdrawal associated with some prescribed medicines: An evidence review*. Public Health England.

Taylor-Page, C. (2022, September 3). Top 10 myths about the critics of psychiatry. *Mad in the UK*. www.madintheuk.com/2022/09/critical-psychiatry-what-do-critics-believe/

Timimi, S. (2021). *A straight talking introduction to children's mental health problems* (2nd ed.). PCCS Books.

Tinghog, P., Hemmingsson, T. & Lundberg, I. (2007). To what extent may the association between immigrant status and mental illness be explained by socioeconomic factors? *Social Psychiatry & Psychiatric Epidemiology, 42*(12), 990–996.

Tseris, E. (2020). *Trauma, women's mental health and social justice*. Routledge.

Tuke, S. (1813). *Description of the retreat*. Society of Friends.

UNHRC. (2019). *Report of the Special Rapporteur on the right of everyone to the enjoyment of the highest attainable standard of physical and mental health*. (2019) UNHRC Document A/HRC/41/34. UNHRC. https://digitallibrary.un.org/record/3803412?ln=en

van Dorn, R.A., Swanson, J.W., Elbogen, E.B. & Swartz, M.S. (2005). A comparison of stigmatizing attitudes toward persons with schizophrenia in four stakeholder groups: Perceived likelihood of violence and desire for social distance. *Psychiatry: Interpersonal and Biological Processes, 68*(2), 152–163.

Varese, F., Smeets, F., Drukker, M., Lieverse, R., Lataster, T., Viechtbauer, W., Read, J., Van Os, J. & Bentall, R. (2012). Childhood adversities increase the risk of psychosis: A meta-analysis of patient-control, prospective- and cross-sectional cohort studies. *Schizophrenia Bulletin, 38*(4), 661–671.

Ventimiglia, I. & Seedat, S. (2019). Current evidence on urbanicity and the impact of neighbourhoods on anxiety and stress-related disorders. *Current Opinion in Psychiatry, 32*(3), 248–253.

Walker, I. & Read, J. (2002). The differential effectiveness of psychosocial and biogenetic causal explanations in reducing negative attitudes toward 'mental illness'. *Psychiatry: Interpersonal and Biological Processes, 65*(4), 313–325.

Watson, J.B. & Rayner, R. (1920). Conditioned emotional reactions. *Journal of Experimental Psychology, 3*(1), 1–14. http://psychclassics.yorku.ca/Watson/emotion.htm

Wetterberg, L. (1999). Melatonin and clinical application. *Reproduction, Nutrition, Development, 39*(3), 367–382.

Wilkinson, R. & Pickett, K. (2009). *The spirit level: Why more equal societies almost always do better*. Allen Lane.

World Health Organization (WHO). (2001). *World Health Report 2001*. WHO.

World Health Organization (WHO). (2019). *International classification of diseases (11th rev.) (ICD-11)*. WHO.

World Health Organisation (WHO). (2021). *Guidance on community mental health services: Promoting person-centred and rights-based approaches*. WHO. https://www.who.int/publications/i/item/9789240025707

Wright, A., Jorm, A.F. & Mackinnon, A.J. (2011). Labeling of mental disorders and stigma in young people. *Social Science & Medicine, 73*(4), 498–506.

Zubin, J. & Spring, B. (1977). Vulnerability: A new view of schizophrenia. *Journal of Abnormal Psychology, 86*(2), 103–126.

Further reading and resources

Books

Anyone interested in critiques of the current mental health system will find all the other books in the *Straight Talking Introduction* series, published by PCCS Books, essential reading:

A Straight Talking Introduction to Being a Mental Health Service User, by Peter Beresford (2010).

A Straight Talking Introduction to Children's Mental Health Problems (2nd ed.), by Sami Timimi (2020). A highly recommended critique of current psychiatric practices with children and young people that takes a strongly non-diagnostic perspective.

A Straight Talking Introduction to Psychiatric Drugs: The truth about how they work and how to come off them (2nd ed.), by Joanna Moncrieff (2020). In an updated and rewritten second edition – an accessible, hard-hitting scrutiny and critique of the evidence for the 'chemical imbalance' hypothesis on which psychiatric drug prescribing is based and the effects of these drugs.

A Straight Talking Introduction to Diagnosis (2nd ed.), by Lucy Johnstone (2022). Also now in an updated second edition, a sharp critique of psychiatric diagnosis and the flawed evidence on which these diagnoses and the medical model of mental 'illness' are based.

A Straight Talking Introduction to the Power Threat Meaning Framework, by Mary Boyle and Lucy Johnstone (2020). Outlines a new framework for understanding and supporting people experiencing acute and severe mental distress that looks to the wider social and environmental factors, rather than individual impairments or dysfunction.

We also recommend:

A Manifesto for Mental Health: Why we need a revolution in mental health care, by Peter Kinderman (Palgrave Macmillan, 2019). A professor of psychology proposes a radical new way of organising and running our mental health system.

Accepting Voices, edited by Marius Romme and Sandra Escher (Mind, 1993). A ground-breaking book about learning to live with voices.

Agnes's Jacket: A psychologist's search for the meanings of madness, by Gail Hornstein (PCCS Books, 2012). Gail Hornstein's meetings with, and reflections on, people who challenge accepted views about madness.

Anatomy of an Epidemic: Magic bullets, psychiatric drugs, and the astonishing rise of mental illness in America, by Robert Whitaker (Crown Publishing Group, 2011). A compelling overview of the research on psychiatric drugs demonstrating that, overall, they cause more disability than they cure.

The Assault on Truth: Freud and the seduction theory, by Jeffrey Masson. (Farrar, Straus & Giroux, 1984).

Attachment Theory and Psychosis, Katherine Berry, Sandra Bucci & Adam Danquah. (Routledge, 2019). A guide to using attachment theory to assess, formulate and treat psychosis-related problems.

Beyond Belief: Alternative ways of working with delusions, obsessions and unusual experiences, by Tamasin Knight (Peter Lehmann Publishing, 2013). Offers a new way of helping people deal with unusual beliefs by encouraging supporters to consider working within the person's belief system. Downloadable free from www.peter-lehmann-publishing.com/books/knight.htm

Can't You Hear Them? The science and significance of hearing voices, by Simon McCarthy-Jones (Jessica Kingsley, 2017).

Coproduction: Towards equality in mental healthcare, edited by Julian Raffay Don Bryant, Pamela Fisher, Mick McKeown, Catherine Mills and Tim Thornton (PCCS Books, 2022). A powerful call for involvement of service users as equal partners in policymaking and the design and delivery of mental health services.

Cracked: Why psychiatry is doing more harm than good, by James Davies (Icon Books, 2013). James Davies' extraordinary expose of how the *DSM* is created, featuring interviews with past and present members of the influential committees that have produced its several editions.

Crazy Like Us: The globalisation of the Western mind, by Ethan Watters (Constable & Robinson, 2011). A hard-hitting look at the damaging effects of exporting the Western diagnostic model of mental health across the world.

De-medicalising Misery: Psychiatry, psychology and the human condition, edited by Mark Rapley, Joanna Moncrieff and Jacqui Dillon (Palgrave

Macmillan, 2011). An inspiring collection of essays about non-medical approaches to distress.

Doctoring the Mind: Why psychiatric treatments fail, by Richard Bentall (Allen Lane/Penguin, 2009). A thorough, research-based overview of currently available psychiatric interventions and their limitations.

Drop the Disorder! Challenging the culture of psychiatric diagnosis, edited by Jo Watson (PCCS Books, 2019). Psychologists, counsellors, psychotherapists and users and survivors of mental health services critique psychiatric diagnosis and explore alternatives and how it can be challenged. An empowering read.

Experiencing Psychosis: Personal and professional perspectives, edited by Jim Geekie, Patte Randall, Debra Lampshire and John Read. (Routledge, 2011). Examines first-person accounts alongside current research to suggest how personal experience can contribute to professionals' attempts to understand and help.

Formulation in Psychology and Psychotherapy: Making sense of people's problems (2nd ed.), edited by Lucy Johnstone and Rudi Dallos (Routledge, 2013). A comprehensive overview of formulation-based practice.

Inside Out, Outside In: Transforming mental health practices, edited by Harry Gijbels, Linda Sapouna and Gary Sidley (PCCS Books, 2019). Showcases pioneering projects offering user-centred, non-medical, trauma-informed ways of helping people experiencing mental distress and crisis.

Living with Voices: 50 stories of recovery, edited by Marius Romme, Sandra Escher, Jacqui Dillon, Dirk Corstens and Mervyn Morris (PCCS Books, 2009). Fifty people describe how they have overcome their problems with hearing voices outside of the illness model by overcoming feelings of threat and powerlessness and discovering that their voices are not a sign of madness but a reaction to problems in their lives.

Lost Connections: Why you're depressed and how to find hope, by Johann Hari (Bloomsbury, 2018). Journalist Johann Hari takes a fascinating journey through what we know about depression, based partly on his own experiences of diagnosis and psychiatric drugs.

Madness Contested: Power and practice, by Steven Coles, Sarah Keenan and Bob Diamond (PCCS Books, 2013). A readable collection of essays looking at criticisms of and alternatives to current mental health practice.

Making Sense of Madness: Contesting the meaning of schizophrenia, by Jim Geekie and John Read (Routledge, 2009). An exploration of subjective experiences of psychosis and what it means to those who experience it.

Mental Health, Race and Culture (3rd ed), by Suman Fernando (Palgrave MacMillan, 2010). Psychiatrist Suman Fernando critiques psychiatry from the perspective of non-Western cultures.

Models of Madness: Psychological, social and biological approaches to psychosis, edited by John Read and Jacqui Dillon (Routledge, 2013). A comprehensive overview of critiques of all aspects of psychiatric theory and practice.

Our Encounters with Madness, edited by Alec Grant, Francis Biley and Hannah Walker (PCCS Books, 2011). An edited collection of 36 service user and carer accounts of diagnosis, personal experience, and the mental health system. The stories are frank, varied and uncensored.

Psychology, Mental Health and Distress, edited by Dave Harper, John Cromby and Paula Reavey (Palgrave MacMillan, 2013). A textbook for student practitioners in mental health, offering a balanced, holistic approach.

Psychosis: Stories of recovery and hope, edited by Hannah Cordle, Jerome Carson and Paul Richards (Quay Books, 2010). Fifteen people tell their stories, and professionals describe various approaches to understanding and helping, including the traditional medical model as well as the recovery approach.

Sanity, Madness and the Family by R.D. Laing and Aaron Esterson (Tavistock Press, 1964). A classic account from the 1960s, showing family dynamics behind the diagnosis of 'schizophrenia.'

Searching for a Rose Garden: Challenging psychiatry, fostering mad studies, edited by Jasna Russo and Angela Sweeney (PCCS Books, 2016). A collection of racial critiques of the psychiatric system from the perspectives of those forced to use them and recovering from them

Sedated: How modern capitalism created our mental health crisis, by James Davies (Atlantic Books, 2021). Explores the links between capitalism, politics and the drug industry to explain how and why prevalence of mental health problems has continued to increase year on year, despite the supposed benefits of modern psychiatry.

Sky-diving for Beginners: A journey of recovery and hope, by Jo MacFarlane (Scottish Independent Advocacy Alliance, 2014). Jo MacFarlane's moving account of her journey to recovery. Available from edinburghjo@yahoo.co.uk

Stabilisation pack. A range of self-help guides produced by service users and the psychology team in Cwm Taf University Health Board, to help people who are experiencing reactions to trauma and provide advice on managing these symptoms. https://cwmtafmorgannwg.wales/services/mental-health/stabilisation-pack/

Tales from the Madhouse: An insider critique of psychiatric services, by Gary Sidley (PCCS Books, 2015). Clinical psychologist Gary Sidley reflects on his career as a nurse working in the mental health system and calls for change.

The Body Keeps the Score: Mind, brain and body in the transformation of trauma, by Bessel van der Kolk (Viking, 2014). A thoughtful and encouraging explanation of the impact of trauma on our minds and bodies, setting the foundations for the trauma-informed approach by one of its leading proponents.

The Genetics of Schizophrenia, by Colin Ross (Manitou Communications, 2020).

The Myth of Mental Illness, by Tomas Szasz (Harper & Row, 1961). Another classic account from the 1960s, challenging the idea that there are such conditions as 'mental illnesses'.

The Practical Handbook of Hearing Voices: Therapeutic and creative approaches, edited by Isla Parker, Joachim Schnackenberg and Mark Hopfenbeck (PCCS Books, 2021). Chapters from survivors and users of services and practitioners setting out a wide range of non-medical approaches to working with voices, drawing on the Hearing Voices Network model.

The Spirit Level: Why equality is better for everyone, by Richard Wilkinson and Kate Pickett (Allen Lane, 2010). Influential and accessible analysis of the effects of economic inequality on our mental wellbeing and the clear links with social and economic inequality

They Say You're Crazy: How the world's most powerful psychiatrists decide who's normal, by Paula Caplan (Da Capo, 1996). A classic critique of the process of diagnosing people, from a US perspective.

This Book Will Change Your Mind About Mental Health: A journey into the heartland of psychiatry, by Nathan Filer (Faber & Faber, 2019). Former mental health nurse Nathan Filer tells the stories of people diagnosed with 'schizophrenia' in this accessible exploration of current debates in mental health.

Toxic Psychiatry: Why therapy, empathy and love must replace the drugs, electroshock, and biochemical theories of the 'New Psychiatry', by Peter Breggin (Fontana, 1993). One of the earliest and most powerful critiques of psychiatry, by a US psychiatrist.

Trauma and Recovery: From domestic abuse to political terror, by Judith Herman (Basic Books, 2015). Another classic – a profound and moving account of the role of trauma in all our lives, from the personal to the political.

Trauma, Women's Mental Health and Social Justice, by Emma Tseris (Routledge, 2020). A discussion of how mental health services have responded to women's trauma.

Understanding Mental Health and Distress: Beyond abnormal psychology, edited by John Cromby, David Harper and Paula Reavey (Palgrave Macmillan, 2013). The first UK undergraduate textbook to be co-authored with service users and based on a non-diagnostic perspective.

Understanding Psychosis and Schizophrenia (revised ed.), edited by Anne Cooke (British Psychological Society, 2017). An accessible publication for psychologists that opens up new ways of understanding and working with experiences labelled as psychosis and 'schizophrenia'. Free from www.understandingpsychosis.net

Users and Abusers of Psychiatry: A critical look at psychiatric practice (classic edition), by Lucy Johnstone (Routledge, 2022). A re-issue of this classic text offering an accessible overview of the limitations of current psychiatric practice. Updated with a new introductory paragraph from the previous edition in 2000.

Blogs

Discursive of Tunbridge Wells. Articles and interviews on a range of mental health topics. **https://blogs.canterbury.ac.uk/discursive**

Laura Delano. Laura Delano's website and blog tells the story of her recovery from 13 years in the psychiatric system. **www.lauradelano.com**

Psychiatry through the looking glass. *Psychology Today* blog series by John Read. **https://www.psychologytoday.com/gb/contributors/john-read-phd**

The blog that shouldn't be written: Madness, trauma and recovery. Campaigner and survivor of psychiatry, Indigo Daya tells her story. **www.indigodaya.com**

Websites

A Disorder for Everyone! Videos, talks, articles and resources supporting the 'A Disorder for Everyone' events that challenge traditional psychiatric theory and practice. **www.adisorder4everyone.com**

Behind the Label. Rachel Waddingham is a former service user, now a writer and trainer. Her website has links, articles and resources.
www.behindthelabel.co.uk

Council for Evidence-Based Psychiatry. Supports the evaluation and use of best evidence to inform best practice in mental health, and hosts articles and resources on its website. **www.cepuk.org**

Critical Mental Health Nurses' Network. A group formed to promote critical thinking about the practice, culture and environment of mental health nursing. **https://criticalmhnursing.org/about-us**

Critical Psychiatry Network. A network of more than 350 psychiatrists, two thirds of whom are based in the UK, the rest spread around the world, who take a broadly critical perspective on current psychiatric theory and practice. **www.criticalpsychiatry.co.uk**

Dolly Sen. Dolly Sen is an award-winning writer, artist, performer, filmmaker and activist for change in the mental health system. **www.dollysen.com**

Dr Terry Lynch. GP Dr Terry Lynch challenges the medical model of depression in his courses and resources. **www.doctorterrylynch.com**

Emerging Proud. Resources, support and personal stories for people who see their crises in spiritual, mystical or transcendent terms. **www.emergingproud.com**

Fireweed Collective. Offers mental health education and mutual aid through a healing justice and disability justice lens and seeks to disrupt the harm of systems of abuse and oppression often reproduced by the mental health system. **https://fireweedcollective.org**

Hearing Voices Network. Offers information, support and understanding to people who hear voices and those who support them. It also aims to promote awareness, tolerance and understanding of voice hearing, visions, tactile sensations and other unusual experiences. **www.hearing-voices.org**

I Got Better. A collection of videos by people who see themselves as having recovered. **www.igotbetter.org**

Inner Compass Initiative. Extensive collection of resources about psychiatric drugs and how to withdraw from them. **www.theinnercompass.org**

Intervoice. The website of the International Hearing Voices Network (the International Network for Training, Education and Research into Hearing Voices). It includes extensive international resources about ways of overcoming the difficulties faced by people who hear voices, as well as the more positive aspects of the experience and its cultural and historical significance. **www.intervoiceonline.org**

International Institute for Psychiatric Drug Withdrawal. Supporting the process of withdrawing from psychiatric drugs through practice, research and training. **www.iipdw.org**

Jacqui Dillon. Trainer, writer and voice-hearer Jacqui Dillon's website. **www.jacquidillon.org** She also describes her experiences of rejecting psychiatry at **www.youtube.com/watch?v=JHzHliy5yeQ**

Mad in America. An invaluable resource for critical perspectives on all aspects of mental health. Includes inspiring blogs by a number of former service users who are now activists and campaigners. **www.madinamerica.com**

Mad in the UK. One of Mad in America's sister sites, hosting a UK-oriented collection of blogs, news, articles and resources. There are also 'Mad in….' sites in Asia Pacific, Brazil, Canada, Sweden, Finland, Italy, Norway and Spain. **www.madintheUK.com**

Mental Health and Survivor Movements and Contexts. A fascinating compilation from numerous perspectives of the history of the service user/survivor movement, including personal accounts.
http://studymore.org.uk/mpu.htm

Mind Freedom International. Mind Freedom aims to 'win human rights campaigns in mental health, challenge abuse by the psychiatric drug industry, support the self-determination of psychiatric survivors and mental health consumers and promote safe, humane and effective options in mental health'. The website also has a large collection of personal stories.
www.mindfreedom.org and www.mindfreedom.org/personal-stories

National Paranoia Network. Website with ideas and resources for people experiencing suspicious thoughts and paranoia.
www.nationalparanoianetwork.org

Paranoid Thoughts. Clinical psychologist and self-help book author, Daniel Freeman hosts this website about 'unfounded or excessive fears about others'. Includes first-person accounts by people who have experienced suspicious thoughts and paranoia. www.paranoidthoughts.com

Paula J. Caplan. Articles, books and links by the late Paula Caplan, US psychologist and leading campaigner against psychiatric labels, who died in 2021. www.paulajcaplan.net

Power, Threat, Meaning Framework. The main Power Threat Meaning Framework website, supporting this new way of understanding and working with experiences labelled as 'psychiatric illness' – hosts articles, blogs, resources, videos and good practice examples.
www.bps.org.uk/power-threat-meaning-framework

The Voices in My Head. An inspiring TED talk by psychologist and voice hearer Eleanor Longden describing her own experience of voice hearing and the psychiatric system, and how she survived.
www.ted.com/talks/eleanor_longden_the_voices_in_my_head

Voice Collective. Hosted by Mind in Camden, a resource 'for young people who hear, see and sense things others don't'.
www.voicecollective.co.uk

Name index

A
Abramson, L. 107
Ahn, W. 67
Ahriman 16
Ainsworth, M.D.S. 97
Ajax 17
Albee, G. 119, 139–140
Alexander, F. 16, 17, 23
Alloy, L. 107
American Psychiatric Association (APA) 8, 10, 14, 34, 44, 45, 51, 53, 56, 77
Angermeyer, M. 61, 64
Appignanesi, R. 96

B
Bandura, A. 102, 103
Barker, C. 62
Barry, M. 61
Beavan, V. 77
Bebbington, P.E. 80
Beck, A. 89, 104, 107
Bell, S.M. 97
Bentall, R.P. 32–33, 54–55, 132, 134
Blehar, M.C. 37
Boerhaave, H. 23
Bourdieu, P. 57
Bower, P. 61
Bowlby, J. 96–97
Boyle, M. 14, 127, 131
British Psychological Society (BPS) 56, 128, 131
Brody, D.J. 46

Brown, P.M. 67
Bullimore, P. 61
Burdett, J. 120
Burton, R. 22
Bush, G. 29

C
Cahalan, S. 54
Cain, A. 34, 44
Carter, L. 67
Cash, A. 99
Cassels, A. 44
Cervantes 22
Cervone, D. 97
Champagne, F. 33
Clements, J. 33
Cooper, M. 111
Copeland, J.R.M. 54
Cosgrove, L. 44
Cozolino, L. 65
Cromby, J. 15, 34, 52, 70, 77, 99, 104, 105
Curley, J. 33

D
Darwin, E. 23
Davies, E. 80, 120
Davies, J. 33, 44, 57
Degenhardt, L. 41
Descartes, R. 11
De Wattignar, S. 34, 44
Dietrich, S. 61

Dillon, J. 61
Dilsaver, S.C. 37
Ducey, C. 18, 19

E
Eaton, W. 72
Einstein, A. 105
Ellis, A. 104
Emperor Constantine 20
Equality Trust 73

F
Falret, J.-P. 25
Felitti, V. 80
Ferenczi, S. 95
Fonagy, P. 97
Fortney, J. 72, 117
Foucault, M. 15, 24
Frances, A. 56
Freud, S. 18, 27, 89–96, 108
Friedli, L. 24
Fromm, E. 95
Fromm-Reichman, F. 94–95
Furnham, A. 60–61

G
Geekie, J. 61
Greenberg, J. 95
Greene, S. 61
Griffiths, A. 130
Gu, Q. 46
Gumley, A. 86

H
Haaga, D. 107
Hahn, P. 31
Hahn Le Quan-Bui, K. 38
Hall, W. 41
Hamilton, S. 30
Harper, D. 56, 66, 105
Harrison, G. 72
Harrop, C.E. 41
Haslam, N. 67
Haslem, J. 23
Heald, A. 46

Health and Social Care Information Centre 46
Healy, D. 44
Hearing Voices Network 12, 136
Herron, W.G. 54
Hills, P. 104
Hippocrates 17–19
Hollingshead, A.B. 71
Holzinger, A. 62
Husserl, E. 108

I
Institute of Psychiatry 80
Ishtar 16

J
Janowsky, D.S. 37
Janssen, I. 76
Jenkins, T.A. 39
Johnson, B. 132, 133
Johnson, R. 81
Johnstone, L. 14, 49, 127–128, 131
Joint Commission on Mental Illness and Health 67
Joseph, J. 31, 116
Joshi, S. 73
Jung, C. 94

K
Kakaje, A. 81
Karanci, A. 64
Khalifeh, H. 81
Kierkengaard, S. 108
Kirk, S.A. 10
Kirsch, I. 47
Kirschenbaum, H. 111
Klein, D. 116
Kohn, M. 71
Kraemer, M. 21
Krimsky, S. 44
Kutchins, H. 10
Kvalle, E.P. 66, 67

L
Larkin, W. 46, 78, 81

Larkings, J.S. 67
Lebowitz, M. 67
Lee, C. 8
Liu, Q. 114
Longden, E. 66
Lorenz, K. 96

M

Mad in America 87
Magliano, L. 62, 64
Martinez, A.G. 56
Maslow, A. 107, 108
Masson, J. 17, 28, 33, 94, 95
McBride, O. 132
McCabe, R. 62
McCartney, G. 72
McGill, C. 65
Michelet, J. 21
Miller, N. 16, 17
Moncrieff, J. 14, 18, 35–36, 38, 39, 44, 46, 83, 117, 137
Morgan, C. 86
Morrison, A. 46, 78, 81
Mortensen, P. 73
Moses 16–17
Mosher, L.R. 44
Moskowitz, A. 46
Moynihan, R. 44
Mullen, P. 79
Murray, R.M. 136–137

N

National Alliance for the Mentally Ill (NAMI) 64

O

OECD 46
Open Dialogue 136

P

Pake, M. 104
Pariante, C. 18
Pavlov, I. 99
Pederson, C. 73
Pervin, L. 97

Pickett, K. 73–75, 140
Pilgrim, D. 60
Pilkington, P.D. 61
Pinel, P. 24–25
Pistrang, N. 62
Plato 18, 19
Porter, R. 15
Priebe, S. 62
Proteus 17
Public Health England 72
Pūras, D. 135

R

Rampello, L. 37, 116
Rayner, R. 28, 99
Read, J. 14, 17, 18, 28, 29, 30, 31, 33, 34, 35, 36, 44, 46, 47, 56, 59, 60, 61, 62, 63, 64, 65, 66, 67, 68, 72, 73, 76, 77, 78, 79, 80, 81, 83, 86, 87, 104–107, 134–135, 137
Reavey, P. 105
Redlich, F.C. 71
Rees, J. 60
Reil, J. 25
Risch, S.C. 37
Rogers, C.R. 89, 108–111
Rogers, D. 60
Romme, M. 61
Rose, S. 32, 47–48
Rosen, G. 16, 17
Rosenhan, D. 54
Rosenthal, N.E. 37, 54
Ross, C. 31
Royal College of Psychiatrists 45, 133
Rush, B. 23
Ryan, C. 8

S

Sagayadevan, V. 65
Sampson, L. 76
Sanders, A. 30
Sanders, P. 88, 109, 140
SANE in the UK 64

Schatzberg, A. 116
Schizophrenia Society of Canada 64
Schlenger, W.E. 77, 81
Scull, A. 24
Seedat, S. 76
Selesnick, S. 16, 17, 23
Shakespeare, W. 22
Sharfstein, S. 44
Shevlin, M. 42, 80, 133–134
Shiva 16
Shooter, M. 44
Simon, B. 18, 19
Skinner, B.F. 27, 28, 98, 100–101
Slater, L. 54
Soteria 136
Sprenger, M. 21
Spring, B. 32
Srinivasan, T.N. 64
Stansfield, S.A. 72
Stearn, R. 24
Storr, A. 96
Sullivan, H.S. 95
Suokas, K. 72
Sweeney, A. 126–127

T

Taylor, J. 77
Taylor, S. 46, 72,
Taylor-Page, C. 57
Thara, R. 64
Thase, M.E. 44
Timini, S. 53
Tinhog, P. 77
Trower, P. 41
Trump, D. 132
Truss, L. 132
Tseris, E. 77
Tuke, S. 24
Tuke, W. 24–25

U

United Nations 44
United Nations Human Rights Council (UNHRC) 135

V

van Dorn, R.A. 62
Varese, F. 46, 80
Ventimiglia, I. 76

W

Walker, I. 66
Watson, J.B. 27, 28, 98, 99
Wettergerg, L. 37
Weyer, J. 22
Wilkinson, R. 73–75, 140
World Health Organization (WHO) 14, 44, 47, 96, 136, 139
Wright, A. 56

Z

Zarate, O. 96
Zubin, J. 32

Subject index

A
A-B-C model 104
abuse 7, 14, 70 (*see also* childhood abuse, violence, women)
adolescents 40, 79
adverse childhood experiences (ACEs) 80
alcohol 35–36, 40, 412, 63
   problems 72, 87, 101, 114
alienists 25
all-or-nothing thinking 2106
antidepressants 46–47, 62, 72, 77, 137
anxiety 11, 18, 31, 35, 38, 70, 76, 77, 92, 110, 114, 115, 133–134
   disorders 52, 72, 78, 79, 80
   social, 36, 135
attachment theory 96–98, 119, 126
'attention deficit hyperactivity disorder' (ADHD) 51, 53
austerity 24

B
behaviourism 27, 98–99, 100–101
bereavement (*see also* loss) 13, 83
biological
   factors 12, 29, 31, 42, 59, 60–67, 116–117, 138
   psychiatry 4, 63, 67, 68, 86
   theories 2, 18–19, 25, 44, 52, 138
biopsychosocial model 31–32
brain
   and biology 34–35
   chemical imbalance 37–39, 52
   disease 30, 66
bullying 7, 8, 9, 67, 80, 117, 122–123

C
cannabis 40–42, 75
   and psychosis 41–42
causes of mental distress
   external, 117
   internal, 118–129
childhood
   abuse 13, 31, 33, 46, 59, 63, 78–79, 87, 117, 121, 122–123, 137, 138
   neglect 13, 24, 31
   sexual abuse 42, 77, 95
Christianity 20
classical conditioning 99–100
cocaine 40, 75
cognitive theory 86, 103–107, 118
computerised axial tomography 29
conditional love 109, 110
confinement 23–24
   The Great Confinement (Foucault) 24
conscious, the 92, 93
cortisol 11
Covid-19 46, 132, 133, 134
   Psychological Research Consortium Study 132–134
culture 76, 83, 89, 90

D

'Decade of the Brain, The' 29
depression 8, 13, 31, 34, 47, 77, 93, 114–116
   cognitive theories and, 100, 118
   formulation and, 120–123, 124
   genetics and, 116
   and grief 82–83
   and neurochemicals 38–39, 118
   non-biological causes 61–62, 72–73, 76, 79, 81, 116–118
   and serotonin 35, 37, 39, 116–117
   and trauma 77–78
diagnosis 14, 51, 53, 57–58
   critiques 135–137
   and ethnicity 767–77
   and formulation 114–116
   'science' of, 53–56
Diagnostic and Statistical Manual of Mental Disorders (DSM) 52, 114, 130
   critiques of, 56
   DSM-III-R 10
   DSM-IV-TR 44, 83
   DSM-5 14, 44, 51, 56, 83
diagnostic model 130
discrimination 9, 65, 76–77, 117, 122–123, 130, 136
disease-centred model 35–36
disturbing behaviour (*see also* behaviourism) 9–10, 12, 16–19, 50, 53, 81, 127, 135
Dogmatists 18
dopamine 36, 37, 40
dreams 81, 90, 94, 122
drug/s
   -centred model 36–37
   companies (*see also* 'pharmaceutical industry') 34, 44, 46, 47, 52, 59, 64, 66, 68, 82, 130
   problems 73, 77, 79
   psychiatric, 130, 131, 134
      prescription rates 46

E

eating disorders 77, 79, 114
economic
   hardship 60, 69
   power 15, 129
ECT 77, 137
ego 92
   defences 92, 93
   super-, 91
environment (*see also* 'nurture') 28, 29–30, 32, 33, 83, 102, 116, 139
   social, 31, 32, 60, 137
epigenetics 33
ethnicity (*see also* race) 9, 76–77

F

family 31, 32, 43, 59, 60, 61, 62, 83, 86
   abuse of children 78
   attitudes, 63–65
   culture 90
   role in mental health problems 69–70, 81, 121–122
   support of, 117, 121
formulation (*see also* PTMF) 113, 120–123
   client's, 123–124

G

gambling 30, 52
   addiction 101
generalised anxiety disorder (*see also* anxiety) 52, 72
genetic
   counselling 33
   predisposition 30–31, 32, 33, 52, 72, 86, 116, 134
      beliefs in, 60, 64, 67
   theories 28, 47

H

habituation 134
hallucinations 61, 77

Hôpital Général (Paris) 22, 24, 71
Human Genome Project 29
humanistic theory 89, 107–111, 118
hysteria 19

I

id 91–92, 94
illness model (*see also* 'medical model') 10, 63, 64, 65, 68
inequalities, socio-economic 131
Inquisition, the 21

L

labels/labelling 9, 50, 57, 138
  harmful effects of, 53, 55
  psychiatric, 50–52, 129–130
language 25, 51–52, 89, 129
learning theories (*see also* 'social learning theories') 98–103
loss (*see also* bereavement) 5, 30, 31, 59, 62, 70, 82–86, 110, 114, 117, 121, 122–123, 133, 138
  of hope 55, 122

M

magnetic resonance imaging (MRI) 29
magnification and minimisation 106
major depressive disorder 114
Malleus Maleficarum 21
masochistic personality disorder 10
medicalisation of life 28, 82, 135
medical model of mental illness (*see also* 'illness model') 10, 17, 27, 63, 83, 117, 135, 136, 137
melatonin 37
Middle Ages, the 20, 21
modelling 103
moral treatment 24–25
morphine 40

N

narrative (*see also* PTMF) 128, 130, 131

nature–nurture debate 16, 21, 27–31, 32–35, 43
neurochemical malfunction 37–39
neuroimaging 29
neurotransmitters 30, 37, 61, 84, 116
norepinephrine 37, 116

O

observational learning 102, 103
obsessive-compulsive behaviour 38, 105
Old Testament 16, 17
operant conditioning 99, 100–102
overgeneralisation 106

P

paroxetine 35, 38
perpetuating factors 120, 121–123
personalisation 106
person-centred therapy 89, 108–111
pharmaceutical industry (*see also* 'drug companies') 28, 43–45
placebo 47
post-traumatic stress disorder (PTSD) 77
poverty 24, 31, 33, 46, 59, 70, 71–73, 76, 77, 82, 117, 121–123, 136
power
  economic, 15, 129
  ideological, 25, 129–130
  imbalance 109, 130, 135
  of language 50
  political, 20
  social, 139
Power Threat Meaning Framework (PTMF) 127–132
precipitating factors 120–121, 122, 124, 138
pre-conscious 92
predisposing factors 120–121, 122
prejudice 55, 56, 65–68
preventative factors 120–121, 122
projection 93,

Prozac 47
psychoanalysis 89–98
psychosis (*see also* 'schizophrenia') 29, 62, 70
   cannabis-induced, 40–43
   and childhood adversities 43, 72, 80
   Freud on, 94
   and loss 86
   and violence 81

Q
Quaker values 24

R
race (*see also* 'ethnicity') 17, 76
rape 77, 78, 80–81, 117
   war-, 81
rational emotive behaviour therapy 104
reaction-formation 93
reason 17–19, 20, 22, 28
   Age of, 23
receptor sites 38, 41
reinforcement 28, 101, 103
reliability (research) 53–57
religion 15–17, 20–22, 23, 28
Renaissance 22
repression 93
resilience 134
right to health (*see also* UNHRC) 135

S
'schizophrenia' 3, 30–31,
   as brain disease 34, 35, 67
   diagnosis 54–55
   genetics of, 30, 33
   prejudice and stigma 65–68
   psychosocial causes (*see also* child abuse, family, gender, loss, poverty, stress. trauma, urbanicity, violence) 46, 59, 60–63, 67, 71–72, 137

science 6, 11, 22–23, 90
   social/behavioural, 27–28, 71, 98, 126
seasonal affective disorder (SAD) 37
selective abstraction 106
self-medication 43,
self-structure 110
serotonin 35, 37, 38–39, 67, 116–117
sexuality 8, 10, 90, 93, 109
Skinner box 100
social (*see also* biopsychosocial)
   control 18
   factors 3, 18, 21, 23, 24, 29, 31–34, 55, 60, 62–64, 66, 69, 72, 73, 76, 77, 86, 136, 137
   isolation 9, 76
   justice 95, 131, 139–140
   learning theory 102–103, 119
   media 79
   norms 15, 129
   science 27, 126
social anxiety disorder 36, 135
social worker 10
stigma/tisation 8–9, 55, 56, 67, 81, 130
   de-, 66, 68
   self-, 67
stress 11, 59, 60–62, 64, 69–70, 86–87, 116, 119, 122–123,
   post-traumatic, 77, 133
   -vulnerability 31–32
sublimation 92
suicide/ality 8, 78–79, 81, 85, 93
   research 87
super-ego 91

T
Talmud, the 17
trauma 30, 32, 42–43, 60, 61, 64, 66, 69–70, 77–81, 110, 120, 125, 127, 130, 134
   -informed approaches 126–127, 129
traumatic stress 133
tryptophan 38–39

U

unconditional acceptance 109
unconscious 88, 90–94, 98
unemployment 30, 31, 36, 42, 72, 76, 117, 122–123, 130, 136
United Nations Human Rights Council (UNHCR)
Right to health report 135
urbanicity/isation 73–76

V

validity (*see also* reliability) 53–55
vicarious learning 103
violence 20, 22, 31, 46, 70, 73, 78, 80–81, 122, 136
  against children 77, 117
  against women 10, 77
  partner-, 77
voluntary behaviours 100

W

wellbeing 140
  psychological , 134
women
  abuse 78, 79, 81
  diagnosis/treatment rates 77, 137
  prescribing rates 46, 77
World War II 96, 104
World Health Organisation (WHO)
  Guidance on community mental health services 136

Y

York Retreat 24

Also by PCCS Books

The *Straight Talking Introductions* series
edited by Richard Bentall and Pete Sanders

---

*A Straight Talking Introduction to the
Power Threat Meaning Framework*
Mary Boyle and Lucy Johnstone

*A Straight Talking Introduction to Psychiatric Drugs:
The truth about how they work and how to come off them*
Joanna Moncrieff

A Straight Talking Introduction to Psychiatric Diagnosis
Lucy Johnstone

*A Straight Talking Introduction to Children's
Mental Health Problems*
Sami Timimi

*A Straight Talking Introduction to Being a
Mental Health Service User*
Peter Beresford

**Available at discounted prices with free UK postage from
www.pccs-books.co.uk**